Bio Chemi

With

Repertory

B. JAIN PUBLISHERS (P) LTD

USA — EUROPE — INDIA

BIOCHEMIC POCKET GUIDE WITH REPERTORY

9th Impression: 2018

Published by Kuldeep Jain for
B. JAIN PUBLISHERS (P) LTD.
D-157, Sector-63, NOIDA-201307, U.P. (INDIA)
Tel.: +91-120-4933333 • *Email:* info@bjain.com
Website: **www.bjain.com**
Registered office: 1921/10, Chuna Mandi, Paharganj,
New Delhi-110 055 (India)

Printed in India by
J.J. Offset Printers

ISBN: 978-81-319-0536-4

CHARACTERISTICS OF THE 12 SALTS

Medicine	Condition of Tongue	Condition of Discharge	Generally suited to people born during
Calc. Fl.	Hard, or cracked or flabby tongue.	From Nose: Lumpy, yellow, or thick. Ulcers and fistula: Thick yellow pus. Menses: Flooding during the period.	21st June to July 22nd.
Calc. Ph.	Bad disgusting taste in the morning—Tongue swollen or blistered.	Discharges like white of an egg.	Dec. 21st to Jan. 21st.
Calc. Sul.	Tongue coated as if with dry clay; sore taste, sometimes soapy acrid.	Yellow purulent-occasionally mixed with blood.	Oct. 23rd to Nov. 22nd.
Ferr Phos.	Tongue clean, red (sometimes dark red). Inflamed or swollen.	Haemorrhages—bright-red stools or vomiting contain undigested food.	Feb. 20th to March 21st.
Kali Mur.	Blisters or ulcers on tongue; white or greyish white coating on tongue.	White as a rule—sometimes yellow.	May 21st to June 21st.

Medicine	Condition of Tongue	Condition of Discharge	Generally suited to people born during
Kali Phos.	Brownish, mustard coloured dry or inflamed—Offensive breath.	Diarrhoea with painless thin stools-rice water colour—carrion like odour. Dysentry with putrid bloody stools. Blood thin, blackish, with offensive odour.	March 21st to April 21st.
Kali Sulp.	Yellow, slimy, at times with white edges; Insipid taste; or taste lost;	Yellowish, Slimy, or greenish mucus discharge (Puls).	Aug. 23rd to Sept. 23rd.
Mag. Phos.	Generally clean; whitish in diarrhoea.	Menses-Dark flow; Diarrhoea-watery	July 23rd to Aug. 22nd.
Nat Mur.	Loss of taste; frothy saliva on the sides; or Dry tongue with sensation of an hair; Sometimes salty taste.	From all mucus membranes there are excessive thin watery secretions; Catarrh with thin watery discharge or with loss of smell and taste; watery discharge from eyes; Involuntary loose stools with dryness of mouth. Thin watery vomitings. Thin menstural flow; Leucorrhoea thin; watery, smarting.	Jan. 21st to Feb. 20th.

Medicine	Condition of tongue	Condition of discharge	Generally suited to people born during
Nat. Phos.	Moist, creamy, golden yellow coating at the back part of the tongue. Acid, or coppery taste.	Eyes; Golden yellow discharge. Ears: Scabs with yellow discharge. Acid Sour Vomitting, particularly in morning. Diarrhoea—Jelly like green—sour smelling, slimy, watery, purulent stools. Leucorrhoea : Acrid discharge ; yellow, watery, causing itching, rawness and soreness. Perspiration ; sour smelling. Eczema : Yellow secretion smelling acrid.	Sept. 23rd to Oct. 22nd.
Nat. Sulph.	Bitter taste, greenish brown, or grey coating. Burning blisters on the tip of tongue.	Nose : Pus changes to green when exposed to light. General billiousness ; green discharges ; Yellowish green discharges in gonorrhoea. Menses ; Profuse with diarrhoea in morning. Yellowish secretion from Eczema.	April 21st to May 21st.

Medicine	Condition of tongue	Condition of discharge	Generally suited to people born during
Silicia	Induration of tougue ; ulcers	Nose : Corriding discharge ; offensive, thick, yellow, Heptic eruptions around nostrils ; Diarrhoea with offensive discharges; Painful piles ; fishure or fistula in anus Gonorrhoeal discharges thick; yellow.	Nov. 22nd to 21st Dec.

The Theory of Biochemical Treatment

THE body is made up of cells. Different kinds of cells build up the different tissues and organs of the body. The difference in the cells is largely determined by the kind of inorganic salts which enter into their composition. If we burn the body, or any part of it, we obtain the ashes. These are the inorganic constituents of the body, the salts of iron, magnesia, lime, etc., which build up its tissues. Besides these inorganic salts, the body is composed of water and organic substances in the proportion of one-twentieth of inorganic salts to the remainder of water and organic matter; but the latter is inert and useless in the absence of the inorganic cell salts. These are the real tissue builders, the architects of the organism, and both the structure and vitality of the body depend upon their proper quantity and distribution in every cell. The biochemical treatment uses these inorganic cell salts, when properly perpared for assimilation, and they are the Tissue Remedies, capable of curing every curable disease and ameliorating most incurable ones.

Health is the state of the body when all the cells composing the various tissues are in a normal condition, and they are kept in this state when they each receive the requisite quantity of the needful cell salt required for the upbuilding of the different tissues.

Disease is an altered state of the cell produced by some irregularity in the supply to the cells of one of the inorganic tissue salts. Imperfect cell action results, diseased tissues and organs follow, and all the phenomena of disease are developed. Now the cure consists in restoring the normal cell growth, by furnishing a minimal dose of the inorganice substance whose molecularmotion is disturbed, which disturbance caused the diseased action. To do this successfully, it is necessary to know what salts are needed for the up building of the different tissues and for their normal action. This knowledge is derived from physiological chemistry, and hence this treatment of disease by supplying the needed tissue salt is called the biochemical treatment.

What is more rational, what is more natural, founded as it is on natural law, that where there is a deficiency in one or more of the component parts of the constituents of an organism, that this deficiency will produce a deranged or a diseased condition; or, more logical, than by the supplying of these lacking elements an equilbrium will again be restored, and the organism returned to its normal condition.

By giving a tissue remedy in such a dose as can be assimilated by the growing cells, the most wonderful and speedy restoration to healthy function is brought about in every case of curable disease. All disease that are at all curable are so by means of the tissue remedies properly prepared to the needs of the organism. This is very important, and one it depends the success of the treatment, just as much as on the correct selection of the particular cell salt. It seems reasonable that, to make the cell salts immediately useful, they should be prepared in the same delicate form in which nature uses them, and that if they are absorbed by the microscopic cropuscles, they must themselves be finer than the corpuscles. We know that the mineral or cell salts are infinitesimally subdivided in the different kinds of food we take, thus capable of assimilation by the cells.

THE DIFFERENT CELL-SALTS.

The cells of each tissue group receive their own special and peculiar cell salt ; for instance, those entering into the promotion of nerve cells are Magnesia, Potash, Soda and Iron; of bone cells, Lime, Magnesia and Silica, etc. etc., which are, as a rule, extracted by the body from the food we take.

There are twelve Tissue Remedies—the twelve inorganic salts found in the ashes of the body, all essential to the proper growth and development of the body. They are the

	Of Lime, Calcarea phosphorica.
	Of Iron, Ferrum phosphoricum.
Phosphates	Of Potash, Kali phosphoricum.
	Of Soda, Natrum phosphoricum.
	Of Magnesia, Magnesia phosphorica.

	Of Potash, Kali muriaticum.
Chlorides	Of Soda, Natrum muriaticum.
	Of Lime, Calcarea sulphurica.
Sulphates	Of Soda, Natrum sulphuricum.
	Of Potash, Kali sulphuricum.

Fluoride of Lime, Calcarea fluorica ; and Silicic Oxide, pure flint or Quartz, Silica.

Of these those, entering into the formation of nerve cells, and hence useful as remedies in diseases of the nervous system, are Magnesia., phos., Kali phos, etc.; of muscle cells, the same and Kali mur.; of bone cells, Calcarea, Silica, etc., etc.

FREQUENCY OF DOSE.

Dose—Two to four tablets.

In acute conditions, a dose one to two hours apart; in severe or painful affections, a dose every ten to fifteen minutes; for chronic cases, from two to four dose daily, as may be required.

ABSCESS.

Treatment—Application of heat, poultices of flax-seed or linseed. When the abscess has opened, the wound should be bathed with warm *Succus Calendula*, one part to five, and after wards a cloth with some *Calendula Cerate* be applied.

Remedies—Ferrum phosph., every hour, when there is much redness, pain and throbbing in the parts.

Calc. sulph. when matter has formed ; this will assist the maturing of the abscess and in many cases render opening the abscess unnecessary.

Silica—After the abscess breaks, this remedy should be used. It ripens the abscess and promotes suppuration, rendering it healthy.

ACIDITY.

Treatment—Avoid the free indulgence of starchy foods, potatoes, mushes, puddings, etc.

Remedies—Natrum phosph. is the chief remedy.

Calcar. phosph. may be given in the same way, morning and night, as a constitutional remedy to permanently cure the gastric weakness giving rise to acidity.

ACNE.

Treatment—Look to diet, avoid fat and rich food. Proper attention to bathing, exercise and the bowels is necessary. If there is any menstrual disorder, see to that.

Remedies—*Natrum mur.* 12x trituration; a dose night and morning should be given to persons with bad, earthy complexion, who are bloodless and inclined to be consitpated and generally depressed in body and mind.

Kali mur. 6x three times a day, for pimples on face and neck, especially after errors in diet—pimples filled with thick, white matter.

Calcar phos.—Especially during time of puberty. Menses are apt to be rather too early and too free in young girls; much backache

AMENORRHEA.

Treatment—Nourishing food, plenty of outdoor exercise, salt water baths. Avoid too much school work and home study.

Remedies—*Natrum mur*. 12x —A dose night and morning, in chlorotic and anemic girls, who are depressed mentally, have a sallow complexion and are inclined to be constipated.

Calcar phosph. 6x—Same dose may be given after *Natrum mur* has been taken for one month.

Kali phos. 6x may be given when, in consequence of the menstrual disturbance, bronchial and lung troubles appear, and the patient is depressed, languid and weak.

Clinical Cases—1. Case of a young girl whose menses had not appeared for several months, and who began to have chest difficulties as a consequence thereof. *Kali phos.*, dose night and morning. The menses soon reappeared, and in four weeks she had no more chest pains.

2. A girl, aet. 22, who always and scanty menses, which, during the past year, had completely ceased, and caused head and eye troubles, received, May 12, 1887, *Kali phos.*, six powders. After using it six days the menses reappeared with violent headache and lasted seven days, and her other troubles gradually disappeared. (Monatsblatter.)

Dr. George Royal reports a case of amenorrhoea with the following symptoms. cured with *Kali phos. 3x*: "Constant dull headache, drowsy all day, cross and snappish; criese asily so fidgety she could not control herself."

ANEMIA.

Treatment—Avoid the excessive use of iron Good nourishing food, warm clothing and out-door exercise are of much benefit.

Remedies—Calcar phosph. 3x. two tablets three times a day. This remedy acts by supplying new blood-cells. Waxy appearance of skin, headache, ringing in ears, vertigo, cold extremities, tendency to profuse menstruation.

Ferrum phosph. 3x follows the above as soon as improvement of the general health sets in. There is a lack of red blood in the system, pale lips, blue rings under eyes, tendency to cough, headaches.

Natrum mur. 12x, two tablets three times a day is especially useful in young girls with dirty complexion, who have frequent palpitation, are blue and melancholy, have bad dreams, constipation, backache and symptoms of malaria—such as chills, feverish turns, perspiration, neuralgia, etc.

Clinical Cases—Dr. S. Powell Burdick furnished us with two cases of anæmia, both in young ladies, æt, 19 and 21. Both presented the following characteristic symptoms: Pale, anæmic countenance great exhaustion, depression of spirits, violent attacks of frontal headache extending to the occiput. The youngest had suffered from this condition for six or seven years. and received treatment from several physicians, homœo pathic and allopathic, receiving from the latter large quantities of iron, without any benefit whatever. The eldest had also been anæmic for several days. All their symptoms were promptly relieved, the color returning even to rosy cheeks; the ears, which were formerly pale and almost translucent, became reddish and natural in color. The remedies employed were first *Calcarea phos.*, for ten days or two weeks, followed by *Ferrum phos.*, for two weeks, then returning to the *Calcarea phos.* again. About six months sufficed to cure permanently in each case.

ANGINA PECTORIS

Remedies—Magnesia phops. 6x.

Kali phoph. 6x, night and morning may be given occasionally to ward off the attacks.

APPETITE. LOSS OF.

Treatment—Avoid the use of tonics, containing drugs and spirits. Plenty of fresh air and moderate exercise and bathing in salt water should be enjoyed. Sec that the bowels are in a good condition.

Remedies—Kali phosph.—Nervous weakness, gone feeling, palpitation.

Calcar. phosph., when there is much flatulence, acidity. Especially useful after any acute illness or when associated with any drain on the system.

ARTHRITIS

Ferrum phos.—At the commencement this remedy should be given in repeated doses when there are febrile symptoms present, and later on in the disease it may be given as an intercurrent. The joints are painful on moving, motion sets up and increases the pain. **Tenalgia crepitans.**

Kali mur.—In acute arthritis, for the swelling or when the tongue is coated white. It may be alternated with *Ferrum phos.* Movement aggravates the pains. It is useful especially after *Ferrum phos*. Tenalgia crepitans.

Nutrum mur.—Chronic arthritis, joints crack (if, tongue and other symptoms correspond acts probably by increasing the eliminations of the urate of sodium). Synovitis, gout, sore hamstrings (verified).

Natrvm mur—Acute gout (after *Ferr. phos.*). Chronic gout, profuse, soursmelling sweat. Rheumatic arthritis, especially of finger joints. Urine dark red. Pains go suddenly to heart; sore hamstrings. It seems to have also a marked effect in hot painful swellings of the knee joint.

Magnesia phos. :—Useful as an intercurrent remedy for the pains (violent). The keynote is excruciating pains, spasmodic in character.

Kali sulph.—In rheumatic arthritis where the pains shift from one joint to another, aggravated by heat. Shifting and wandering rheumatic pains in the joints. Fungoid arthritis. Tumor albus, white swelling.

Silica.—Suppuration of the joints.

Calcarea sulph.—Suppurative process in the joints.

Natrum sulph.—In acute cases (attacks) of gout. This remedy should be alternated with *Ferrum phos.* In chornic gout it alone suffices. Gout in the feet, acute and chronic. Rheumatic arthritis, especially in joints of fingers, pains suddenly go to heart, urine dark-red.

Calcarea phos.—Rheumatic gout worse at night and in bad weather. Hygroma patellæ. Hydrops genu.

Calcarea fluor. Gouty enlargements of the finger-joints.

ASTHMA

Remedies—Ferrum phos. and *Magnesia phos.*, in alternation every 1/4 or 1/2 hour, when there is much wheezing, nausea and lose cough.

Eradicative Treatment—Natrum sulph. 12x, a dose night and morning, especially for children who suffer with asthmatic attacks after some skin disease, eczema, etc., who wheeze up at every change of weather. Give for a few weeks, then substitute *Calcar. phoph.* 3x, to be given in the same way. By persevering for a time with these constitutional remedies, many cases of Asthma can be cured.

Clinical Cases—Female, married, æt. 36, asthma, attack violent, greenish, purulent expectoration, a loose evacuation immediately on rising for past two days; *Natrum sulph.* every two hours. Was enable to lie down that night, respiration and cough much improved and expectoration easier. Next day practically well.

ATROPHY (Marasmus)

Remedies—Calc. phos. 6x, 12x—This is the chief remedy. Diarrhoea, flatulence passes with stools, undigested stools, slow dentition, bones ill-developed.

Kali phos. 6x—General atrophy, particularly of the bones. Fatigue, sleeplessness. Offensive discharges.

Nat phos. 3x, 6x—Marasmus of bottle-fed babies swollen abdomen, enlarged liver, undigested food passes with stools, which smell sour.

Nat. Mur. 6x, 12x—Rapid emaciation of the upper part of the body; child irritable and constipated.

Silica 6x, 30x—Head large but body thin; much perspiration; irritable; offensive footsweat; aversion to mother's milk; stools watery and offensive; slow in learning to walk; fats well yet emaciated.

BACKACHE.

Remedies—Calcar. phosph. 6x. a dose three times a day. Backache in small of back in the morning, numbness coldness and creeping sensation. Backache in young people who grow rapidly and after any exertion.

Natrum mur. 12x, night and morning for backache, relieved by lying on something hard.

Kali phosph. if connected with loss of vital fluids and nervous disturbances generally.

BARBER'S ITCH.

Kali mur. 6x, a dose three times daily alternated with *Calcar sulph.* will cure rapidly. At the same, the beard should be cut off, bathe parts with hot water to which some carbolic acid solution has been added (10 drops to a cup), and afterwards apply some carbolic cerate.

BED WETTING

Remedies. Ferr. phos. 3x, 6x—If inflammation is present, muscular weaknesses.

Kali phos. 6x, 12x—For nervous, highly strung children.

BILIOUSNESS.

Treatment—Persons subject to biliousness should not eat too much meat, drink plenty os water, avoid coffee and high living and take plenty of exercise.

Remedies—Natrum sulph. 6x, every three hours; coated tongue, sallow skin, yellow eyeballs, soreness in region of liver, flatulence.

Kali mur; if caused by eating rich food.

Nutrum phosph; if the tongue is coated with bright yellow fur.

BITES.

Remedies— Nat. Mur 3x, 12x; Relieves the pain; may be used externally and internally.

BOILS (See Abscess).

Accessory Treatment—Foment with hot water, and then poultice with fresh linseed-meal or bread and milk, applying linenrags soaked with *Calendula* lotion afterwards. (For medical treatment. see *Abscess.*) The diet should be in accordance with the condition of patient; if of full habit and living freely, a spare diet may be advisable; but if, on the contrary, the system is a little below par, a more generous regimen should be adopted.

BRAIN-FAG.

Remedies—Kali phosph. 6x, a dose in the morning, and *Silica* 12x, a dose at night, used persistently, will be found the the most effective remedies. They will restore sleep, appetite, confidence, and strength. It may be necessary to follow with *Calcar. phosph.* 6x, a dose before every meal, especially if there is a good deal of general coldness or a tendency to night sweats.

BRONGHITIS.

Treatment—A warm, equable temperature of 70 degrees should be kept in the room, and the patient put to bed. Liquid diet : milk, gruel stewed fruit may be given. In chronic bronchitis, a dry, warm climate will prove very beneficial.

Remedies—Ferrum phosph. 6x. It should be continued twenty-four hours, and if the cough then gets loose, pain and fever less, *Kali mur.* may be alternated with it every two hours. This treatment will generally suffice. *Kali sulph* may be substituted when the cough gets very loose and there is much rattling of much in the chest. A tablet of the 6x. may be given every two hours. The chief remedies for chronic bronchitis are *Kali sulph.*, *Calcar phos.*, and *Silica.* Give one remedy three times daily for one week, then change to another. If improvement shows itself continue the remedy in a higher trituration, and not so frequently.

BUNIONS.

Medicinal Treatment—Silica is an efficacious remedy. *Dose*—Two tablets dry on the tongue, once a day for a week, then wait three days and repeat.

Accesory Treatment—Apply *Arnica* lotion (one tea spoonful of the tincture to four or five tablespoon fuls of water) by means of a linen bandage over the part, especially if there is much inflammation and pain. All pressure mnst be avoided. An *Arnica* bunion plaster may be applied to the enlargement. In some cases it may be necessary to paint the bunion with Iodine.

BURNS AND SCALDS.

Treatment—(1) Cover the burn immediately with cotton wool, to exclude the air ; or the same object (2), cover with linen rags, or cotton wool saturated with olive oil ; or (3) powder the wound plentifully with flour, it keeping well covered by new applications if necessary ; it (4) cover the whole with a plaster of soap, made by scraping white curd soap, and working it into a salve with tepid water, and spreading it upon linen or muslin. Slight or superficial burns or scalds may be relieved by holding the part to the fire, or by applying spirits of turpentine, brandy or spirits of wine to them. In dressing burns, puncture the blisters and remove the old skin, but expose the wound as little as possible to the action of the air ; do not dress oftener than once a day, do not disturb the parts by washing them. The exclusion of the air from the part affected is of the utmost importance. *Calendula Succus* is excellent locally as are also wet applications of *Sulfax.* Internally, give *Ferrum phosph.* 6x.

CANCER OR MALIGNANT TUMOR.

Treatment—Nothing is more certain than that remedies can influence the development, and sometimes cures, growths ; but it requires patience and the physician's skill. The Tissue Remedies are frequently of great use in the treatment of all forms of tumors. Among those of undoubted value are *Calc. fluor., Silica, Calc. phosph.,* and *Kali sulph.*

Calc. fluor—Knots, kernels, etc., in the breast; hardened glands ; hard swelling anywhere. Give one tablet of the 3d trit. night and morning ; after a week, give the 6th, and later the 12th, in order to get the full action of the drug. The other remedies may be substituted and used intercurrently.

Kali phosph.—For the pains of cancer, aud for the offensive discharges.

CARBUNCLE.

Treatment-Keep up the strength of the patient by nourishing food. Poultice with flaxseed dress with aqueous. *Calendula lotion* When healing is commenced, apply *Calenaula cerate.* Internally, use treatment recommended under "Abscess." Whatever remedy is given should be alternated with *Kali phosph.* 6x tablets, one tablet every two hours.

CATARRH.

Treatment—Regulate the diet ; keep the bowels opon; insist upon; maintaining a healthy action of the skin by daily sponging and friction ; insist upon wool being worn next the skin night and day, summer and winter ; insist upon well ventilated sleeping apartments open windows the year round ; teach the patient to breathe through the nose and to fully expand the chest, and have him practice lung gymnastics until he does this properly; and have him live in the open air as much as possible.

As a currative and prophylactic agent in nasal catarrh, pure air is the best topical application and also the best general tonic.

Kali mur--Drynees and stiffness of nose. Hawking of mucus form the back part of the throat. The most satisfactory remedy to begin treatment. Give one tablet every 3 hours. After a week follow it with.

Calcarea phosph., which is especially useful in chronic catarrhal conditions. Nose seems swollen or is ulcerated. The patient takes cold very readily. This remedy has a decided tonic action on the mucous membrane and may be used inter-currently with other remedies that may be indicated. Give one tablet after meals and at bed time.

Natrum mur. is the best remedy when the discharge is thin and watery. "Running colds" are frequent. Cold sores on lips. Loss of smell and taste. Chronic catarrhs in bloodless patients who have much backache and headache.

Kali sulph. is the remedy when the secretions are yellow, slimy.

Natrum sulph., when there is profuse secretion of greenish mucus. After influenza, and when the patient is worse from dam weather.

Silica may be required in very obstinate cases, where the discharges are offensive or where there is a painful chronic dryness of the nose, or plugs in the nose or ulceration of the mucous membrane. This may be followed by *Calcar. fluor.*

CATARHAL FEVER.

Treatment—The most effectual means of relief is good nursing in a moderately warm and equable temperature—a warm bath, or immersing the feet in hot water, and promoting perspiration by a hot bed and warm drinks. Animal food and stimulating drinks must be abstained from. If there is a liability to catch cold, do not at once when coming from the cold air, endeavor to get warm by approaching a hot fire, but do so by degrees. Use plenty of cold water daily over the chest, shoulders, throat and neck, sponging freely for two or three minutes, and applying a rough towel or flesh brush afterwards until well warmed.

Remedies : *Ferrum phosph* and *Natrum mur.*, one tablet of each every hour alternately. When improvement shows itself, lengthen the interval between the dose.

Calcer phosph., one tablet three times daily for the remaining debility. It will act as a tonic.

CHANGE OF LIFE

Remedies : *Ferrum phosph.*, will benefit the tendency to flashes of heat, sleeplessness, hot spells and cold feet, etc.

Kali phos. for the gone. sinking sensations, the restlessness and nervousness; also for sensations of numbness.

Magnes. phos.. for abnormal palpitations, pains, etc.

CHESE AFFECTIONS (See Bronchitis, Pleurisy, etc.).

For pains in chest the best general remedy is *Ferrum phos.*

Dose of the selected remedy—One tablet three times a day, or oftener for more acute attacks.

CHICKEN POX.

Ferrum phos. and *Kali mur.* are the only remedies required. It is not necessary to give many doses, as the disease is mild and runs a short course.

CHILBLAINS.

Remedies : *Calco phos.* 3x, 6x—This is the principal remedy.

Kali mur. 6x, 12x—Useful where there is much swelling.

Ferr. phos. 3x, 12x—In alternation with Kali mur. for the pain and inflammation.

Kali phos. 6x, 12x—To be given inturcurrently to counter the effects of the irritation.

Calc fluo. 6x, 12x—Useful, if there are cracks in the skin.

Kali sulph. 3x, 6x—Broken chilblains exuding thin, yellow fluid.

CHOLERA.

Ferrum phos.—In the first stage, for the vescular disturbances, alternating with *Kali phos.* Cholera infantum discharges frequent, watery, even bloody; child is greatly reduced, falls into stupor, red face, dilated pupils, rolling of head and soft, full-flowing pulse, cholera from checked perspiration.

Kali phos.—When the stools have the appearance of rice-water. Collapse, livid, blue countenance and low pulse.

Kali sulph.—Cramps and other symptoms of cholera.

Magnesia phos.—Choleraic cramps. First stage. Watery diarrhoea with vomiting and cramps in calves.

Natrum sulph.—Is, according to Schussler, the remedy for cholera and cholerine.

Calcarea phos.—Cholera infantum. Green diarrhœa in scrofulous children, slimy, watery, undigested and offensive. Thin body, child looks like an old woman.

Clinical Case—Old man attacked with severe vomiting and diarrhœa, cramps in calves and rice-water discharges. *Kali phos.* cured. (Schussler.)

CIRCULATION, FEEBLE.

Treatment—Plenty of exercise in the open air, good, nourishing food, salt water baths, massage, etc.

Ferrum phosph. and Calcarea phosph. one in the morning and other at night, will soon regulate matters, if there is no organic heart trouble present.

GOLD IN THE HEAD (Coryza).

Treatment—See Catarrhal Fever and Catarrh.

COLDS OF INFANTS (Snuffles).

Accessory treatment—A warm bath at 96 degrees before going to bed, or placing the feet in warm water will generally relieve; and if there is much stuffiness, the bridge of the nose may be rubbed with a little simple ointment or sweet oil. Children should not be accustomed to hot rooms, but taken into the open air freely, care being taken that their feet are dry and warm.

Remedies—Same as "Catarrhal Fever."

COLIC.

Treatment—Apply heat to abdomen and be sure that the feet are dry and warm; give an injection of warm water if the bowels have not moved.

Remedies—Magnesia phos. 3x—Flatulent Colic, forcing the patient to bend double; in children the legs are drawn up. Colicky babies when they cry half the time; no interference with nutrition.

Natrum phos. 6x—Colic with symptoms of acidity, sour smelling stools, vomiting or where worms are present. Give one tablet every hour, and when the immediate symptoms are relieved, give one tablet three times a day.

Natrum sulph.—Colic starting in right groin. Flatulent complaints after confinement or during menses. Bilious colic, with bitter taste in the mouth. Lead colic.

CONCUSSION OF THE BRAIN.

Natrum sulph. 6x is of special benefit for the chronic effects of falls upon the head. Give a does at bedtime.

CONSTIPATION.

Treatment—The bowels should be solicited at a regular time every day, even if there is no action; active exercise the must be taken in the open air, and daily friction used over stomach and bowels with the hand or flesh brush. A cold bath, either sitz or shower, or using cold water over the abdomen, should be taken every morning, together with the employment of a coarse towel or flesh glove. Avoid purgatives.

Diet—A change of diet will generally prove beneficial, and care must be taken not to eat too much at a meal, and to let what is partaken of be simple, easy of digestion, and consisting more of vegetable than animal food—brown bread, barely bread, wholesome ripe fruit, baked pears or apples; avoiding salted meats, cheese, rice, highly-seasoned dishes and the like. Cold spring water should be freely partaken of on rising in the morning and between each meal, but very little liquid should be taken at meals. Figs and dates are of benefit.

Remedies—Kali sulph.—Habitual constipation with insipid, pappy taste and yellow slimy coating on tongue.

Natrum mur.—Dry stools, with torn, bleeding, smarting feeling after stool. Stools are hard, dry and difficult to pass. Hemorrhoids, headache and backache accompanying.

Silica—Rectum seems to have lost the power of expulsion, feces recede after having been partly expelled. Constipation of poorly nourished children with pale, earthy face.

Calcar phos.—Costive, hard stools with blood, especially in old people, associated with mental depression, vertigo, headache.

CONSUMPTION OF THE LUNGS (Tuberculosis).

Treatment—Much can be done by careful hygienic, dietetic and climatic measures. Good, nourishing, easily digestible food, fresh air, avoidance of exposures to rapid changes in the weather, warm clothing, all are essential.—Cod-Liver Oil, Maltine, Kumyss, Cream, fresh butter are of benefit and should be provided.

Remedies—These must be selected according to the general symptoms of the patient, character of cough, state of stomach, bowels, etc. Among the chief are.

Calcar. phos.—In the beginning, when there is loss of flesh, hoarseness, suffocating attacks. cough with soreness and dryness of throat, dull aching in the chest, chronic coughs and night sweats with cold extremities.

Calcar sulph.—When the expectoration with the cough is bloody or greenish yellow.

Silica—Nightly paroxysms of cough with tickling in throat, emaciation, profuse night sweats. Offensive foot sweats. Constipation very marked. Much prostration, patient is always cold. This remedy embraces most of the symptoms that belong to the phthisical dyscrasia, consequently it is of great value for the constitutional condition in hereditary cases.

Ferrum phosph.—Should be used intercurrently for colds in patients inclined to consumption—breathing short, oppressed, hurried with heat and feverishness. Hoarseness and cough, usually dry, sometimes bleeding of nose or from lungs. Blood bright red, frothy.

CONVALESCENCE

Remedies—Cals. phos. 3x, 6x—This is the principle remedy to restore the quality of the blood, to aid assimilation and to tone up the system generally.

Ferr. phos. 6x, 12x—This remedy should be given with Calc. phos. to oxygenize the blood.

COUGH.

Remedies Ferrum phosph.—Short, dry cough after colds, sore feeling in chest, feverishness. Of great value in the beginning of any trouble with the respiratory organs, especially in children. Will usually cut short the attack.

Kali mur.—Loud, noisy stomach cough; croupy; hard cough, thick, whitish expectoration.

Kali sulph.—Cough with yellow secretion. Much rattling of mucus in chest. Patient feels worse in warm room.

Magnes. phos.—Spasmodic and whooping cough, worse at night. Dry cough in nervous patients.

Calcar. phos.—Suffocative cough, better lying down. Cough with expectoration of tough, stringy matter.

Natrum sulph.—Cough with sensation of all-goneness in chest. Chest very sore. Thick, yellowish mucus.

CRAMPS.

Magnes. phosph. is the only remedy necessary. Give one tablet of the sixth potency at bedtime for a few nights.

CROUP.

Treatment—Put on a hot compress around the throat, changing it frequently.

Remedies—The chief remedies for this disease are *Ferrum phosph.* and *Kali. mur.*, given alternately every half hour. If the symptoms do not improve after several hours, substitute *Calcarea phosph.* and *Calcarea fluor* every hour. During convalescence, give *Calcar. sulph.* three times a day until complete restoration of health. Use the 6th tablets, dry on the tongue.

CRYING OF INFANTS.

Treatment—See that the child is comfortable in every way—dry and warm—especially the feet and abdomen. Toast the feet by an open fire, if possible; loosen all bands and see that no pins are pricking any part.

Remedies—These should be selected according to the most probable cause as mentioned above. In general use *Calcar.*

phosph., 3x, followed, if necessary, by *Magnes. phosph.* 3x, given in the same way. During the feething period the occasional use of *Calcar. phosph.* will prevent many unpleasant restless and crying spells.

DEAFNESS FROM A COLD.

May frequently be greatly benefited by remedies. Use *Ferrum phosph.* 6x, one tablet, three times a day, to be followed in a few days, if necessary, by *Kali mur.* same dose and preparation.

DEBILITY.

Kali phosph.—When the nervous system suffers most as evidenced by nervousness, sleeplessness, weakness from the least exertion, bodily and mental. Patient is depressed and in a sensitive state. One tablet of the 3rd potency should be given in a cup of hot milk three times a day or oftener if there is also loss of appetite for food generally.

Calcar, phosph.—is often called for in young chlorotic girls, near the age of puberty, when they are very restless and nervous. They want to go away from home, and, when away, want to come back again; they suffer from headache when at school; they develop very slowly; circulation imperfect; ears and nose cold; constant headaches from artificial light, from atmospheric changes—worse on top of the head; debility following exhausting diseases; menses apt to be too early, with faint feeling in the stomach; a feeling of soreness in the back. In anemia of young, rapidy growing people, in women weakened by rapid childbearing, prolonged suckling, or excessive menstruation or leucorrhea, it has wonderful restorative power. Give one tablet of the threes four times a day.

Natrum mur.—In anemic conditions, where the blood is thin and watery; chlorosis, with habitual feeling of coldness in back; skin is dirty, sallow; frequent palpitation; delayed menses; constipation; watery, smarting discharges between periods; terrible sadness, especially during menstruation ; backache relieved by lying on something hard ; the neck is much emaciated, and emaciation continues even while living well. Especially useful after abuse of quinine ; patient shows marked aversion to bread—longing for salt food. *Natrum mur.* is especially the remedy for malarial symptoms. It is best to give it in tablets of the sixth, a dose three times a day.

DENTITION.

Ferrum phosph. is the remedy for feverish turns.

Natrum mur. when the child drools very much.

Magnes phos. if it twitches and has a dry spasmodic cough, also for colicky turns.

DIABETES.

Remedies—Cali phosps. especially after depressing emotions, patient is weak, nervous and restless. Give one tablet of the 3x for one week three times daily, after which substitute the 6th, and later the 12th potency.

Natrum mur.—Great thirst much wasting, and constipation, are the special indications for this drug.

DIARRHOEA (Looseness of the Bowels).

Treatment—For an acute attack, the best plan is to avoid all food for a few hours ; then take mutton broth with barley, or chicken broth and rice, boiled milk, avoiding solid and irritating food of all kinds, as fruit, vegetables, etc. Keep the bowels and feet warm and dry. Rest in bed, if possible.

Remedies—Ferrum phosph., watery stools, or undigested with colicky pain.

Magnes phosph, if the pains are especially severe.

Cali mur., when the stools are bloody or contain much mucus, tongue coated white.

Dose—Of the selected remedy a dose should be given after every evacuation.

For chronic diarrhoea, the best remedies are *Calcar. phosph.* and *Natrum sulph* Give one tablet of the sixth potency alternately night and morning and after every evacuation.

DIPHTHERIA.

Remedies—Ferrum phosph. and *Cali mur.* should be given in alternation every hour. If there is vomiting of watery fluid, give *Natrum mur.* instead.

Cali phosph. corresponds to symptoms of blood poisoning, very offensive discharge and breath. also, for the paralytic states, resulting from diphtheria. A dose every two hours.

If the larynx becomes involved, give at once *Calcar. fluor.* A dose every half hour.

DIZZINESS.

Calc. phosph. 1x. One tablet after meals.

DISCHARGES.

If fibrinous, stringy, gluey, *Kali mur.* If watery, serous, *Natrum mur.* If thick *Kali sulph.* If yellowish, *Natrum phos.*

It does make any difference in the selection of the remedy, whether the discharge be from the nose, throat, ears or pelvic organs, it is the *character* of the discharge which determines the remedy.

DROPSY.

Various dropsical affections can be benefited by the Tissue remedies, but when they are the results of organic diseases, usually heart and kidney or liver diseases, they are signs of deep-seated mischief and of serious import. The principal remedies are *Kali mur.*, *Natrum mur.* and *Kali sulph.*

DYSENTERY (Bloody-Flux).

Remedies—Kali mur. and *Ferrum phosph.* taken in alternation every two hours will generally suffice in mild cases.

Kali phos., when the stools contain mostly blood, are offensive and there is falling of rectum.

EAR, DISEASES OF THE (Earache).

Treatment—Apply heat and give *Ferrum phosph.* A dose every five minutes until relieved.

EARS, HUMMING IN THE

Kali phosph. is the chief remedy.

EARS, DISCHARGE FROM THE

Kali mur., *Silica* and *Calcar. phosph.* are the principal remedies. Give a dose three times a day of one for one week then substitute the next, and so on.

ECZEMA.

Remedies—*Kali mur.*, *Kali sulph.*, and *Natrum mur.* are the chief remedies. Give one tablet of the sixth potency night and morning for one week; then substiiute the twelfth potency, and if no improvement is apparent after two or three weeks, use one of the other remedies in the same way.

EPISTAXIS (bleeding from the nose)

Remedies—*Ferr. phos.* 3x, 6x—Bright red blood, flushed face.

Kali phos. 6x, 30x—Blood dark, thin, great weakness. Epistaxis due to old age or debility.

Application of cold water on the head, the neck and over the nostrils proves beneficial.

ERYSIPELAS (St. Anthony's Fire).

Treatment—Avoid all applications except flour, cornstarch; or, when procurable ripe cranberries. Honey sometimes is also very efficient.

Ferrum phosph. and *Kali mur.* are the principal remedies. Give hourly dose, alternately until the disease is checked. *Kali sulph.* should be given instead, if blisters form *Kali phosph.* may be alternated with it, if there is much nervous disturbance, weakness, restlessness, etc. A dose may be given every hour until improvement shows itself.

EYE, DISEASES OF.

Kali mur.—Affections with discharge of mucus, ulcers of cornea.

Natrum mur.—Muscular asthenopia, neuralgic pains around eye, with much watering of eyes; granulated lids.

Silica—Styes, kernels and indurations of the lids; scrophulous ophthalmia.

The selected remedy should not be given lower than the sixth potency. For chronic affections the twelfth is better. Give a dose night and morning.

FEVER (Simple or Inflammatory).

Treatment—In the treatment of fever the room in which the patient is, should be cool, airy, and well ventilated, and kept at an even temperature of about sixty degrees. The covering to the bed should in general be light, but suited to the feelings of the patient; the linen should be often changed, and the patient may be frequently sponged down with tepid water. The diet must be light, easy of digestion, and unstimulating—barley-water thin gruel, or arrowroot, toast-water or water to allay the thirst; ice-water or ice mav be held in the mouth, and fruits stewed or in most cases also fresh may be allowed. Lemonade is also grateful. Unfermented grape juice and Kumyss are admirable foods in all cases where fever is present.

Ferrum phos. is the only remedy required. Dissolve three tablets of the 3x in half a glass of water and give teaspoonful doses every hour until relief is obtained, then less frequently.

Kali phos.—For nervous fevers, quick irregular pulse, with nervous excitement and much weakness—mouth dry, blisters around mouth, with tendency to delirium.

FISTULA-IN-ANO

Remedies—Calc. Fluo. 12x is useful in chronic cases.

Silica 6x, 12x—Fissures, discharge of pus.

Calc. phos. & Ferr. phos. to be used alternately.

FLATULENCY (Wind in the Stomach or Bowels).

Magnes. phos. and *Calc. phos.* are the principal remedies. Give *Magnes. phosph.*, one tablet of the third potency after meals, and repeat every half hour until better; give *Calc. phosph.* night and morning as a constitutional remedy.

GALL STONE

Remedies. Calc. phos. 3x, 30x—To prevent the formation of new stones in alternation with *Nat. sulph.*

Mag. phos. 3x, 6x—Spasm from gall stone.

Natrum sulph. 6x, 12x—Cannot bear tight clothing around the waist; bilious subjects.

Taking of pure oilve-oil one teaspoonful twice a day is very beneficial.

GASTRIC DISTURBANCES.

Remedies—Kali mur., if due to errors in diet, especially fat. food.

Natrum sulph., if associated with liver symptoms, jaundiced skin, pain in right side, flatulence, diarrhoea.

GLANDS (Glandular Affections).

No class of diseases is more strikingly benefited by the tissue remedies than acute and specially chronic inflammations of the various glands throughout the body. There is usually a scrophulous taint at the bottom to account for the readness with which, from apparently slight causes, the glands will grow painfull and swell. The treatment of chornic cases requires patience and not too frequent change of remedies. *Kali mur.* is the chief remedy for all acute swellings. *Calcar. phosph.* for more chronic cases. Commence with the 2x. Give three doses daily for one week; then give the third, sixth and twelfth potency in the same way. *Silica* for suppurating glands.

GONORRHOEA.

Remeeies. Calc. sulph. 3x, 6x—Bloody and pus like discharges.

Ferrum phos. 3x, 6x—In the most inflammatory stage; acute stage with febrile condition.

Kali. mur. 3x, 6x—It has almost a specific action in gonorrhoea; white discharges. Inflammatory swelling of testicles for suppressed gonorrhoea.

Mag. phos. 3x, 6x—Sharp stitching pain, relief from hot application; stricture from gonorrhoea; sharp pain in the urethra.

Nat mur. 3x, 30x—Chronic gonorrhoea; watery burning discharges; gleet.

Nat. sulph. 6x, 12x—Gleet, greenish yellow discharges.

Silica. 3x, 30x—Chronic cases; pus like offensive discharges; constant chilliness.

GOUT (Arthritis).

Accessory Treatment—The diet must be very spare during the acute symptoms, as thin gruel, bread and milk, light bread puddings, barley water, arrowroot and the like, oranges, roasted apples, grapes, etc. Keep the affected part in such a moderately cool state as to be comfortable to the patient, without being so warm as to aggravate the severity of the attack, or so cold as to check the insensible perspiration. External applications are generally of little use in a case of gout; those which are warm doing no good and those which are cold having a tendency to suddenly check the inflammation, thereby producing harm. *Kumyss* and unfermented grape juice may be used freely. Friction with the fleshrush during convalescence is beneficial, and the limbs and affected parts should be regularly sponged with cold salt watar every morning, and well wiped and rubbed afterwards. The diet, during convalescence, should consist of a little digestible animal food once a day, with eggs, bread etc., but no wines or spirits.

Remedies—The chief remedy is *Natrum sulph.* 6x a dose three times a day. For acute attacks, *Ferrum phos.* every two hours. If the stomach is involved give *Natrum phosph.* every two hours.

GRAVEL.

Whenever there is a sandy sediment in the urine care should be taken to change the diet, avoiding too rich food and drinking plenty of pure water.

The chief remedy is *Natrum sulph.*, a tablet three times a day; but if there is much acidity at the same time give *Natrum phosph.* instead.

GUMS, SCURVY OF THE (Canker of the Mouth).

Treatment—Avoid food that tends to produce acidity, such as sweets, rich food, etc.

Kali mur. 3x—*Natrum mur.* may be given after *Kali mur.* if the symptoms do not improve very rapidly.

HAY FEVER.

Magnesia phos.—Dr. T. C. Fanning rcommended this remedy as the best one we possess to prevent a threatening attack of hay fever from maturing, or to relax the same when it has already set in. If the weather has been sultry, and the patient stuffy during the day, oppressed with short, anxious breathing, the spasm during the night will come unless this remedy be given every hour during the day and through the evening in hot water.

Natrum mur.—Hay fever from suppressed intermittents; craving for salts; least exposure to sun brings on violent coryza with sensation of itching in nasal and lachrymal passages.

Silicea—Itching and tingling in nose and posteriorly at orifice of Eustachian tubes, with violent sneezing and excoriating discharge. Hoarseness, roughness and dryness, with a tickling cough, worse by cold drinks, by speaking and when lying down at night.

HAEMORRHAGES.

Ferrun phosph. generally suffices, especially in children that grow rapidly. Blood is bright red.

Kali mur. when the blood is dark, black, clotted or tough; vomiting of such blood.

Kali phosph. in weak, delicate people, in the aged, and where the blood is blackish, thin, like coffee grounds.

Of the selected remedy a dose may be given every five to fifteen minutes until relief is obtained.

HAIR.

Falling out of the hair is a frequent sequent to fevers, but here the loss is only temporary, and can he stayed by giving *Calcar. phosph.* three times a day. For the loss and thinning of hair not thus connected faithful brushing is a good tonic procedure. Too frequent washing is not to be advised. An occasional dose of *Calcar. fluor.* and *Silica* will be found beneficial.

HEADACHE, CATARRHAL.

From a cold.

Symptoms—The headache is opressive, frequently better in the morning, worse in the evening, the eyes are full of tears, sneezing, dry heat in the nose, some cough, etc.

Treatment—*Ferrum phosph.* will generally be all that is needed. Glve a dose every half hour.

HEADACHE, CONGESTIVE.

From determination of blood to the head.

Symptoms—Fulness and heaviness of the head, accompanied with gidiness, particularly on stooping, throbing and heat, the beating of the arteries on the neck being visible, vomitting as the pain increase; the pain worse on shaking, moving the head, lying down or stooping, sometimes better when standing.

Principal remedy is *Ferrum phosph.*

HEADACHE, NERVOUS.

Neuralgic pains in the head. *(Megrim)*.

Symptoms—The attacks are frequently periodical, the pain is of a tearing, throbbing or hard-aching character, and is often felt on one side of the head only or in a circumscribed spot. The painful part feels sore to pressure; light, noise and mental agitation are intolerable, and the headache is often attended with servere retching or vomitting of bile and mucus.

Treatment—*Kali phosph.* and *Ferrum phosph.* alternatively every half hour during the attacks. Between the attacks give *Natrum mur.* for one week, then *Silica* for one week, and so on alternatively for a time.

HEAD SYMPTOMS.

Ferrum phosph.—Headache from cold, sun exposure ; throbbing pain ; cold relieves the pain ; headache with red face and eyes ; rush of blood to head ; worse from any motion, noise, jar, combing hair, and at menstrual period,

Calcar. phosph.—Headache of school children, especially at about the time of puberty ; head feels cold, bruised, worse from any exposure ; much dizziness ; ill-humor; want of disposition to do anything ; forgetfull, dull.

Kali phosph.—Headache of students and those worn out by fatigue—old people, and after mental emotions ; pain made worse by noise, which irritates ; sleeplessness, weariness, yawning ; pain sometimes relieved by eating ; menstrual headache with hunger ; tongue coated brownish with foul breath ; pain in back of head and across eyes.

Megnesia phosph.—Spasmodic pain ; very severe neuralgic headache ; shooting pains, with sparks before eyes ; headache due to eye troubles ; better from warmth.

Natrum mur.—Headache with constipation, with vomiting with watering of eyes, and with drowsiness ; after loss of animal fluids ; profuse discharges, night sweats, etc. Here follow with *Calcar. phosph.* Chronic and sick headaches ; headache before and during menses, especially in school girls who study hard, are run down ; anemia ; headache commences in the morning, increase towards noon, and gets better in evening.

Natrum sulph.— Bilious headache with bitter taste : bilious diarrhoea : colicky pain, etc. Also for pain in back part of head, at the base of the brain: must go to bed in a darkened room : cannot tolerate noise.

Silica.—Headache from nerve exhaustion ; after excessive mental strain ; nervous, sensitive patients : weakly persons, fine skin, pale face, lax muscles ; imperfectly nourished These respond quickly to this remedy.

HEARTBURN.

Treatment—Avoid all articles of food that you know from experience to disagree with you.

Natrum phosph. is the principal remedy. Give one tablet of the sixth potency after eating. If there is much flatulence give *Calcar. phosph.* in the same way.

HEART, PULPITATION OF.

Calcar. phosph.—Weak heart ; sharp pain around the heart ; palpitation with anxiety, followed by tremoling weakness.

Ferrum phosph.—First stage of all acute, inflammatory diseases involving the heart ; pulse rapid and full : regulates the circulation.

Kali phosph.—Intermittent action of the heart : ill-effects of mental emotions, palpitation, pain, etc.; palpitation from slightest cause ; physical or mental exertion.

Magnes. phosph.—Shooting pain around heart with spasmodic attacks of palpitation.

Natrum mur.—Watery condition of the blood, shown by anamia, dropsical swelling, ready flushing, and pulpitation; construction around heart; fluttering and intermittent pulse.

HICCOUGH-HICCUP.

Treatment—Holding the breath is the most simple, and in many cases the most effective way of stopping hiccough, or drinking a draught of cold water. When it occurs in infants they may be placed to the breast. If subject to this little trouble, attention should be paid to diet, care being taken not to eat too quickly, nor too much at a time.

Magnes. phosph. is the only remedy required.

HOARSENESS.

Treatment—Use plenty of cold water, or cold salt water, and cold sponging, with vigorous friction afterwards. The diet should be plain and simple; take but little meat, and avoid simulants; keep the feet warm, and do not exert the voice.

Drink warm milk and seltzer during an acute attack and take *Ferrum phosph.* and *Kali mur.* alternately every hour. In very obstinate cases take *Cacar. sulph.*

HYSTERIA.

Treatment—Is medical to some extent, but mainly moral and hygienic. Do not show too much sympathy with the patient and her innumerable aches and pain; encourage self control, self forgetfulness; encourage her to take interest in others, to have a mission of some kind. Discourage reading aimless and trashy literature. Avoid excitement of all kinds, late hours, stimulants, tea and coffee, rich food, etc. Build up the general system by simple but nourishing food, aided by unfermented Grape Juice, Malted Milk, Maltine, Kumyss, etc. Regular exercise in open air, judicious use of bicycle riding, driving, swimming, walking with a cheery companion, all tend to restore the lost stability of the nerves.

Kali phosph.—Nervous attacks from intense emotions—feeling of a ball rising in throat; hysterical fits of laughing and crying ; hysterical yawning and spasms ; general nervousness.

Natrum mur., when associated with delaying menses, patient is greatly depressed, sad and weak. All the symptoms are relieved when perspiring freely.

Calcar. phosph., as a constitutional tonic, may be given twice a day in the food.

INDIGESTION.

Treatment—Look to the diet. Avoid whatever he knows from experience to disagree with him, but do not encourage any dietetic theories. Remember what is good for one patient is not necessarily adapted to another, even when suffering with similar symptoms. Every adult ought to know himself better than any one else what kind of food is most likely to agree with him. Usually a mixed diet of simple nourishing food, eaten slowly and well masticated and at regular intervals is better than restriction to some one or two articles. When coffee cannot be taken try Postum, which possesses a good deal of the flavor and taste of true coffee without any deleterious effects.

Remedies—Ferrum phosph.—Pit of the stomach is tender to touch : vomiting; pain after eating; flatulence; loss of appetite: disgust for milk : cannot take meat ; cannot bear tight clothing : thirst for cold water ; desire for stimulants.

Kali mur.—Tongue coated : complaints from rich and fatty food : bitter taste ; liver sluggish, with pain in right side under shoulder.

Kali phosph.—Hungry soon after eating ; gone feeling in stomach ; pain in left side; weakness of heart ; constant pain in a small spot in stomach : great nervous depression.

Kali sulph.—Yellow-coated tongue : sensation as of a load and fulness in the pit of the stomach ; pain in stomach ; waterbrash.

Magnes phosph.—Cramp in stomach; constriction; hiccough; marked regurgitation after eating ; craves sugar; gastralgia.

Natrum mur.—Stomachache with much waterbrash, offensive breath ; bowels constipated ; loss of desire for smoking ; very thirsty ; sour taste ; aversion to bread ; red spots on pit of stomach.

Natrum phosph.—Great acidity; sour risings; moist, creamy coating of the tongue ; stomach troubles from presence of worms ; heartburn; vomiting of dark, coffee-ground fluid.

Natrum sulph.—Biliousness; bitter taste in mouth ; vomiting of bitter fluid ; heartburn ; copious formation of gas, which gets incarcerated in intestines.

Calc phosph.—A course of this remedy is useful in all chronic cases of indigestion; pain after eating; craving for bacon, ham, salted and smoked meats ; pain relieved by eating and raising wind ; almost an infallible remedy for excessive accumulation of gas in the stomach.

Calc. phosph., 1x trituration, a powder given in water helf an hour after eating, is efficacious in non-assimilation of food.

Calc. sulph.—Desirė for fruit, tea, claret and green vegetables.

Silica.—Chronic dyspepsia, with much chilliness ; extreme hunger ; disgust for warm food, and, intolerance of alcoholic stimulants.

INFLUENZA—GRIPPE.

Natrum sulph. is the principal remedy throughout the course of the disease and for many of the after effects.

Calc. phosph. and *Kali phosph.* may be given during convalescence and for the remaining debility.

INTERMITTENT FEVER.

Natrum sulph. is the chief remedy. In the absence of any special symptoms, this will be found the best general remedy. It is especially called for when there are bilious symptoms, yellow complexion, bronze-coating of tongue, bilious bloody stools.

Natrum mur.—Chill is apt to return in morning about 10 O'clock ; great thirst ; headache ; backache; fever blisters; neuragia of head and face.

In order to prescribe successfully for this obstinate disease the conditions between the attacks of chills and fever should be noted, they indicate the curative remedy more likely than the character of the different stages, although these, too, must be included in our estimate of the case.

JAUNDICE.

Natrum sulph. is the chief remedy. Give a dose every four hours. *Kali mur.*, if caused by cold and the tongue is coated whitish.

KIDNEY'S.

Remedies—Ferrum phosph. may be given, a dose every two hours until improvement sets in.

Kali mur. for the dropsical symptoms.

Natrum mur.—Brick-dust sediment ; bloody urine. One of the best remedies alone, or in conjunction with others, in Bright's disease.

Natrum sulph. aids in throwing off gravel by increasing the secretion of urine. Of the selected remedy give a dose three times a-day.

KNEE, SWELLING OF.

May be due to rheumatism or disease of the joint. Any trouble around the knee-joint should be carefully examined.

Kali mur. and *Calcar. phosph.* often act kindly in these affections.

LEGS, CRAMP IN THE.

Sudden contraction of the muscles of the calves of the legs, frequently occurring at night.

The principal remedy for this condition is *Magnes. phosph.*, a dose every quarter of an hour for a few doses. Follow with *Calcar. phosph.*, a dose night and morning.

LEUCORRHEA (Whites).

Calcar. phosph. is the chief remedy, either alone or as an intercurrent remedy ; it acts as a constitutional tonic and is especially useful for young girls. The patient takes cold easily and the discharge is like albuminous mucus. There may be local irritation, itching, etc., of the parts.

Natrum mur—The discharge is watery, irritating, smarting. There may be backache, headache and evidences of impoverished blood.

Kali sulph—Discharge yellow, greenish and thick.

Silica—Leucorrhea takes the place of menses ; patient is cold, very sensitive and constipated. Of the selected remedy give a dose three times a day between the menstrual periods; give one remedy for three weeks, then another if indicated, or substitute *Calcar. phosph.*

LIPS.

The lips are subject to becoming sore, cracked dry, scaly or swollen, or are the seat of a herpetic eruption "cold sores." The best treatment consists in the application of cold cream and the internal use of *Kali mur.* for cold sores, blisters.

Natrum mur. for cracks in the corners of the mouth, or center of lip; sore lips form cold; swelling of upper lip—a dose every three hours.

LIVER AFFECTION.

These are characterized by pain in right side, under right shoulderblade, soreness, bilious symptoms, constipation or loose yellowish stools, etc.

See Gastric Derangements.

Natrum sulph.—Pain in region of liver ; morning diarrhoea; rumbling in bowels; jaundice; bitter taste.

Natrum mur.—Jaundice, with drawsiness, thirst, headache.

Kali mur.—Tongue coated white, from errors of diet, rich, greasy food; cold food, chilling stomach.

LUMBAGO.

Rheumatic pain in the loins.

The treatment consists in application of warmth, friction, porous plaster, and the administration of *Ferrum phosph.*, a dose every hour until relieved.

LUNGS.

The various disease of the lungs require careful hygienic, dietetic and medicinal treatment. The latter may be found almost wholly in the use of the tissue remedies, for just in the treatment of acute and chronic lung diseases they have won their greatest laurels. (See Consumption, Pneumonia, Pleurisy, etc.)

LUNGS, BLEEDING FROM.

The principal remedy required is *Ferrum phops.* Follow with *Calcar phosph.* as a constitutional tonic, a dose three times a day.

MALARIA.

Remedies—Ferr. phos. 3x, 6x—High rise of temperature, vomiting of undigested food.

Kali phos. 6x, 12x—Great debility, profuse sweat.

Nat. mur. 3x, 6x—After the abuse of quinine, great thirst.

Nat. sulph. 3x, 6x—Indicated in all stages, biliousness; fever during rainy season.

MEASLES.

Accessory treatment—The room in which the patient is should be airy, darkened, moderately warm, and perfectly free from draughts, much care being taken that the patient does not catch cold, both during the eruption and for some time afterwards. He may be sponged down frequently with tepid water. The diet should be at first light, afterwards more nourishing; all animal food should be avoided, and all drinks should be given tepid, so as not to chill. Protect the eyes from too strong light. The danger of measles is more in the after effects, especially bronchitis, pneumonia, etc.

The principal remedy is *Ferrum phosph.*, which may be given every two hours, so long as the eruption is not out perfectly, or so long as the cough is troublesome. It may be followed by or alternated with *Kali mur.*, if the tongue is coated, the cough hoarse, glands swollen, more or less deafness. During convalescence give *Calcar phosph.*, a dose every three hours until perfect health is restored.

MEMORY-DEFICIENT.

This is a symptom of advancing age, or it may be temporary in nerve exhaustion, after acute, illeness over-taxed brain.

The treatment consists in cessation from mental labor and the administration of *Kali phosph.*, a dose three times a day.

MENSTRUAL DISORDERS.

Scanty, absent, deficient or checked menstruation,

When suppressed from cold, a chill or sudden emotion, a hot foot-bath, hot drinks and rest in bed will restore the flow. If there is headache, flushing of face, pains, etc.. give *Ferrum phosph*.

Calcar phosph. is the best remedy for scanty menses. Give a dose night and morning between the periods.

MENSTRUATION, PAINFUL.

Magnesia phosph. is the principal remedy and should be given in hot water every quarter of an hour until relieved. Between the periods give *Calcer. phosph.* and *Kali phosph.*, one in the morning and the other at night.

MENSTRUATION, PROFUSE OR TOO FREQUENT.

Causes—Stimulating diet, abuse of stimulants, warm baths, fatigue, compression of the body, sudden emotions, violent exercise, a weakening mode of life, long sickness, excessive nursing of infants at the breats, etc.

Ferrum phosph. is the principal remedy to regulate the flow. Give a dose every two hours or oftener, if very profuse. In the interval between the periods, give it night and morning.

Calcar. fluor. when the system is generally relaxed. It should be given between the periods as above.

Kali mur., if the colour of the flow is dark, thik and coagulated.

Kali phosph., if flow is bright red and offensive.

Natrum mur., if pale and watery. Patient has much headache, backache and is anemic.

Mag. phos.—Worse on right side, relief from heat, too early, flow dark.

· Miss S., æt. 22, brunette, short, plump, round body, large, active brain, intellectual, was since puberty troubled every month with dysmenorrhoea, beginning several hours previous, and during the first day of flow, with severe pains in the uterus, back and lower limbs, and these so severe that they seemed unbearable and hysteria seemed threatening. In one of these attacks I was sent for. Found the patient in bed; the feet has been bathed in hot water and hot cloths applide for hours to the lower abdomen; pains no better. I immediately gave her a large dose of *Magnes. phos.* 6x. In less than half an hour the pains lessened; I repeated the dose; in a few moments the patient was easy, the flow began. and went on the usual time. Next month I advised patient to begin the day before period and take three doses, and on the day period was to come on take a dose every two hours. No pains this month. This process was repeated the third month; no more trouble; patient is now well, and no return of pain for over three years.

MOUTH.

Nursing sore mouth, aphthous sore mouth, consist in the formation of little vesicles on mucous membrane of the mouth, gums and tongue.

Remedies—Kali mur. and *Natrum mur.* are the chief remedies. Dissolve three tablets in a glass half-full of water and give spoonful doses every two hours alternately.

MUMPS.

Treatment—The patient should keep in the house, and avoid exposure to cold and damp ; the glands shou d be fomented with warm water, the face tied up with a handkerchief or piece of flannel. and kept moderately worm. and the diet should be mild and light. If the patient take cold, there is danger of a painful swelling of the testicles.

Remedies—Ferrum phoph. should be given so long as there are any feverish symptoms. a dase every hour. Usually, however, there are none, when *Kali mur.*, a dose every three hours. will be all that is required If the swelling should persist, give a few doses of *Calcar. fluor.*

NECK, STIFF.

Usually the result of cold or rheumatism.

Treatment--See under "Rheumatism." Rub the neck with camphorated oil, wrap two or three folds of flannel or worsted round it, and avoid exposure to cold, draughts of air, or wet. Give *Ferrum phosph.* every two hours.

NERVOUSNESS.

Kali phosph. and *Calcar phosph.* are the principal remedies and should be given as nerve food remedies right along for some time. Begin with the 6x, giving three doses a day of one for one week, then change to the other. If the patient is chilly and very senstive and rather of intellectual turn of mind, give *Silica 6x* night and morning. After one week, change to the 12th and give the same way.

NETTLERASH.

The treatment consists in avoiding irritating foods, keeping the bowels in good condition, bathing the parts with oatmeal water, and giving *Natrum mur.* and *Kali mur.* in alternation every two hours.

NEURALGIA.

Remedies—*Ferrum phosph.* should be given when the face is hot and red and the pains increased on moving the head.

Kali phosph. suits pale, irritable persons and when pains are accompanied with much weakness.

Natrum mur.—Pains that return at a certain time each day or are attended with flow of tears. Constipation is a frequent symptom with *Natrum mur.*

Magnes. phosph.—Pains that come and go very suddenly and are always made better by the application of warmth.

Kali sulph.—For pains that shift a good deal, and when they are better in cool open air, but worse towards evening.

Calcar. phosph.—Pains that are associated with numbness and coldness, and always worse at night and every change of weather.

NIGHTMARE.

Treatment—Let the supper be light; avoid fatigue and heavy bed clothing. Give a dose of *Kali phosph.* before retiring.

NOISES IN THE HEAD.

May be due to recent catarrh of the Eustachian tube, an extension form an ordinary cold, or as a result of too large doses of quinine, etc.

If from a cold, give *Ferrum phos.*, if after quinine, give *Natrum mur.*, a dose every three hours.

NOSE, BLEEDING FROM THE.

Treatment—Immerse the face in the coldest water, and dash cold water, or vinegar and water, up the nostrils, or apply ice or ice-water to the root of the nose, or apply cold cloths or metal to the nape of the neck or back. Keep the head as much elevated as possible, and let the diet be spare and simple in character. As bleeding from the nose often relives congestion, the treatment should be adapted to the urgency of the symptoms, which if slight, need not be much interfered with. Persons subject to nose-bleeding should lead a temperate life, with modirate and regular exercise, a nourishing diet, avoiding stimulants, and should make a free use os cold water.

The principal remedy is *Ferrum phosph.* Dissolve three tablets in a cup of cold water, and give a swallow every few minutes until relieved.

OVARIES.

Pain in region of groin in females about the time of menses is a common symptoms, and usually connected with other menstrual disturbances. Rest, application of heat, and attention to the bowels, are necessary. Internally. give *Kali phos.* and *Magnes. phos.*, alternating every hour. Between the periods. give *Calcer. phos.* night and morning.

PAINS.

Remedies—Ferr. phos. Throbbing pains with heat, inflammation and congestion, strained muscles and tendons, sprains. Pains resulting from cuts and wounds (a little powdered *Ferr. Phos.* should be applied locally). *Ferr. phos.* and *Mag. phos.* are the principal remedies for checking pains.

Mag. Phos. Spasmodic, craming-pains, with acute stabbing, boring sensations, neuralgia, sciatica, menstrual pains, etc.

Kali Phos. Itching of the skin with nervous irritation or crawling sensation chilblains which itch and tingle.

Calc. Fluo. Aches and pains of the legs with feeling of heaviness due to bad circulation. Pains in the lower part of the back with dragging sensation.

Calc. Phos. Deep-seated pains in the bones and joints, severe at night. The pains are allevated by moving the limbs.

Kali Mur. Pains accompanied by soft swellings. tonsilitis, fibrinous discharges. Gastric pains after eating fatty or rich food.

Silica. Pains due to formation of thick, yellow pus, boils, gum-boils, abscesses, etc.

Kali Sulph. Stomach pains with sensation of pressure and fullness at the pit of stomach.

Nat. Mur. Pains accompanied by watery symptoms, pulsations felt all over the body.

Nat. Pohs. Digestive pains with heartburn. sour acid risings.

Nat. Sulph. Pains associated with liver disturbances, notably biliousness, sick heacache, nausea. etc.

PARALYTIC SYMPTOMS.

Numbness and lamenness ; rheumatic paralysis ; loss of sensation or motion in a part, may be relieved by the use of *Kali mur.*, if due to rheumatism ; later, *Calcar. phosph.*, a dose night and morning.

Silica is the remedy, if the condition is due to the suppression of food-sweet, which has freqently coused paralytic conditions and cured only by giving a remedy restoring the occustomed sweat.

PERSPIRATION.

Abnormal, when due to weakness, as after acute illness or general run-down conditions of the body, will be lessened by sponging the body with vinegar and water, or cologne spirits and water, and giving at the same time *Calcar phosph.*, 3x.

PHARYNGITIS.

Redness, pain and swalling of the mucus membrane of the mouth and throat.

Remedies—Ferrum phosph., if the part are dry, hot with painful swallowing ; a dose every hour.

Kali mur., if the tongue be coated white and parts swollen.

Natrum phosph., if the tongue be coated with a yellowish deposit.

The chronic form of pharygitis is often due to smoking, which must be stopped. A course of *Kali mur.*, a dose of the third three times a day, will often work wonders.

PILES (Hemorrhoids).

Treatment—The pain and irritation often present are much relieved by the free application of cold water either by bathing or immersion. *AEsculus Cerate* spread on lint and kept constantly to the parts is sometimes beneficial. When the inflammation is great, rest and the horizontal position should be observed, with a mild vegetable diet. Everything heating, stimulating, and constipating, must be avoided in the general diet, all highly-seasoned food and the like. Individuals subject to piles should bathe in the sea as often as convenient, or in salt water baths. During an attack, injections of cold water may be used daily ; suitable exercises should be taken, and every endeavor made to keep the bowels regular.

In the treatment of piles, attention must be paid to disturbances in the functions of the liver, the digestive organs and the bowels, otherwise a cure cannot be achieved.

Ferrum phosph.—Inflamed and bleeding piles, must be used before the tumors are hardened. Give a dose every hour and bathe with *Hamamelis* extract.

Calcar. fluor. is the chief remedy for the permanent cure. It is useful for blind piles frequently with backache and constipation, etc. After an acute attack, it is the remedy for the remaining tumours. Give one tablet every three hours Use the 6th potency, later the 12th or 30th.

Magnes. phosph. is the remedy, when the piles are exceedingly tender and painful.

PIMPLES (Acne.)

The treatment consists in encouraging healthy elimination through skin and bowels. Eat fruit, vegetables, and drink plenty of fresh water. Thorough washing with soap and water the affected part, then powder with corn-starch, will prove beneficial.

The chief remedy is *Kali mur.* followed by *Calcar. suiph.* Give a dose three times a day.

PLEURISY, FALSE—Rheumatic Pleurisy. Stitch in the Side—(Pleurodynia).

The treatment consists in the application of heat and administration of *Ferrum phosph.* in hourly doses until relieved.

PLEURISY.

Treatment—The patient's room must be kept quiet, moderately warm, but well ventilated. Perfect rest should be observed. All kinds of animal food and heating fluids should be avoided, and the diet should consist of farinaceous articles, barley water, arrowroot, thin gruel, light vegetables, milk, etc.; returning during convalescence to beef-tea, chicken-broth, etc. A wet bandage may be applied over the painful part with advantage or if the pain is severe, hot linseed meal poultices, hot fomentation, etc. During recovery, care must be taken to guard against catching cold.

The principal remedy at first is *Ferrum phosph.* This may be followed by *Kali mur.*, a dose in alternation with *Ferrum* every hour.

PLEURO-PNEUMONIA.

Ferrum phosph., *Kali phos.* and *Kali mur.* are those most frequently indicated. The remedies must be given frequently every hour at least, supplemented by absolute rest, easily assimilated food, milk, broths, etc. The application of poultices may prove of much comfort, but should be done very carefully without disturbing the patient much or exposing him in any way, otherwise they are a delusion.

PREGNANCY.

Remedies—Calc. Phos. 3x, 6x–Menstruation during lactation period ; weakness during pregnancy.

Calc. Fluo. 6x, 12x–Insufficient and weak after-pains ; uterus does not properly and timely contract after childbirth: prolapsus, miscarriage flooding ; failure of milk or scanty supply of milk ; hard knots and lumps in the breasts.

Ferr. Phos. 3x, 12x–Used extensively to avoid post-labor inflammation and fever. Generally prevents the puerperal fevers if given immediately after child-birth. Guards against after-pains, indigestion and vomiting of undigested food.

Kali Mur. 6x, 12x-Constipation, morning, sickness, vomiting of white mucus.

Mag. Phos. 3x, 6x–Weak, short pain, cramps of the legs, puerperal convulsions.

Kali Phos. 6x, 12x–Promotes and excites labour. If given a month previous to cofinement, it facilitates the labour and makes the confinement and labour easier.

RED GUM—Infant Rash.

Bathe the child in bran or oatmeal water, and after thorough drying with a soft towel, powder freely with corn-starch. Give a dose of *Ferrum phosph.* night and morning. If the child is teething, give *Calcar. phosph.*

RHEUMATISM.

Treatment—Keep the parts warm and dry ; flannel underwear is essential. See that the bowels are kept in good condition ; avoid to much meat ; drink milk.

The first remedy in this painful affection is *Ferrum phosph.* It should be given every hour until improvement shows itself. If the joints are swollen, alternate with it *Kali mur.* every two hours. For very violent pains, *Magnesia phosph.* is to be used, a dose every hours, stopping the other remedies meanwhile.

Calcar. phosph. is the remedy when every change of weather brings back rheumatic pains.

Rickets (Rachitis).

The treatment of a rickets child requires careful attention to details. The diet must be regulated ; sugar and starchy food must be curtailed ; Mellin's food, fresh cow's milk, broths, plenty of fresh air ; sunlight and cleanliess must be found in the nursery ; warm clothing, combination flannels, warm shoes and stockings are all very necessary ; massage, salt water baths, inunction of oil are useful aids. A course of the Tissue Remedies will accomplish excellent results.

Calcar. phos. is the principal remedy. The bones are soft ; child is emaciated, sweats profusely, is weak and cold ; may have diarrhoea, sallow, earthly complexion etc. It is best to give it continuously in the food, beginning with tablets of the first or second potency and putting one in all its food ; later, give the third and sixth potency about three times a day. This remedy may be given in alternation with any other that may be indicated.

Natrum mur.—Especially when the neck is very thin and the thighs, also, are much emaciated.

Silica.—Head large, rest of body greatly wasted away ; abdomen swollen, hot; ankles weak; offensive diarrhoea; child very nervous ; sensitive, irritable, cold, tendency to boils ; child feels better when wrapped up very warmly.

Natrum phosph.—This remedy is especially useful for poorly nourished children, when there is much acidity, sour-smelling stools, perspiration, etc. ; stools often clay-colored.

RINGWORM.

The treatment consists in the application of Carbolated Vaseline and the internal administration of *Kali mur.*, a dose three times a day.

ST. VITUS DANCE (Chorea).

Remedies—Magnes phosph. and *Calcar. Phosph.* are the principal remedies. For the acute attacks, give a dose of *Calcar phos.* morning and night, and *Magnes. phos.* every two hours during the day. When improvement sets in, give one dose of each daily, one in the morning and the other at night.

SCARLET FEVER (Scarlatina).

The patient with scarlet fever must be separated. It is contagious from the initial sore throat until the last branny scales have been removed. Six weeks quarantine is not unsual.

SCIATICA.

Remedies—play but a minor role in the treatment. For simple forms, nothing outside of the hourly administration of *Ferrum phos.* is required. For the severe types *Kali mur.*, *Kali phos.* and *Calc. phos.* are beneficial.

A most painful neuralgic affection of the large nerve supplying the leg, often very obstinate and dependent frequently upon constitutional defects. In the treatment, great attention must be paid to the condition of the bowels, as a loaded colon suffices to greatly aggravate the pain, also to the condition of the foot apparel, sometimes heavy shoes or boots, and warm stockings going far to cure an attack.

Cali phos.—Pain down back of thigh to knee, great restlessness, moving about gently gives some relief for a time.

Natrum sulph.—In gouty patients, pain in hip-joint, worse moving about or raising from a seat.

Natrum mur.—Chronic cases. Pains better by heat, worse right side, hip and knee ; hamstrings feel contracted.

Magnes phos.—When the pains are very severe. Given in hot water, it will often mitigate them.

For very obstinate cases *Calc. phos.* and *Silica* may be tried.

Clinical Cases—Mr. B. has been suffering for seven months with sciatica in left leg; the pain was very severe and fast undermining his health; he had been treated by a very skillful physician all this time, and almost every known remedy was tried, until the physician himself gave up the case and said that he could do nothing more. I was called, found patient suffering with a dull, tensive pain, extending the whole length of the sciatic nerve of the left leg, worse on slightest motion; prepared a small power of *Kali phos.* 6x, in half a glass of water, and gave a teaspoonful every ten minutes for an hour, when the pain was much better; patient then slept until morning. Next night the pain returned; gave same remedy, but with no results. The next night gave *Kali phos.*, and very soon the pain was relieved; continued *Kali phos.* every two hours, a small power dry for a week, and then four times a day for a month; once during that time he had a slight attack, which was soon stopped by putting one of the powers in a half glass of water, and giving a teaspoonful every ten minutes for awhile. A year has passed and there has been no return of the trouble. (G. H. Martin, M. D.)

SHINGLESS.

Treatment—Power the parts with corn starch after applying a little vaseline and give *Kali mur.* and *Natrum mur.* in alternation, a dose every two hours. If the pain is severe substitute *Kali phosps.*, a dose every hour.

SKIN DISEASES.

Remedies : *Calc. phos.* 3x, 6x—Suppurative skin diseases; thick yellow discharges.

Kali mur. 6x, 12x—Tick eczematous eruptions; secretion of white pus; warts; milky white coating on the tongue.

Kali sulph. 6x, 12x—Yellow-watery eruption, sticky pus; sudden suppression of eruptions.

Nat. mur. 6x, 12x—Clear watery eruption; eczema from taking too much salts; water secretions; herpes.

Nat. phos. 3x, 12x—Yellow cream like discharges; yellow scabs; milk crusts acidity.

SLEEPLESSNESS (Insomnia).

Is an early symptom of an exhausted condition of the nervous system and should be treated by looking to the general health. Avoid mental work, especially in the evening; stimulants, especially coffee, but see that the patient does not go to bed hungry. Often a cup of beef-tea or hot milk at bedtime will insure a good night's rest. See that the feet are warm when retiring; if necessary, put a hot water bag in the bed.

The best general remedy is *Kali phos.* It may be given with advantage in hot milk on retiring for the night.

Silica may be given during the day, if the patient is nervous and excitable and chilly.

SLEEP, DISTURBANCES OF.

"Mrs. C. says when she has a severe pain in back of neck and head, and so nervous she could not allow any one to talk to her, could not lie still or sleep, one power of *Kali phos.*

would relieve her in a few minutes, and she would sleep as if she had taken morphia, and would feel sleepy for the entire by and night following the dose."

SMALL-POX (Variola.)

Treatment—The patient's room should be cool, thoroughly, ventilated, and darkened; some antiseptic should be used freely, either on cloths dipped in the solutions or in the form of spray. Cool, fresh air should be admitted several times a day, and the patient should lie on a mattress and be lightly covered. The linen should be frequently changed, and the free use of cooling drinks allowed. The diet during the feverish symptoms should be spare and light—barley-water, thin gruel, etc,; and if there is no diarrhea, roasted apples, stewed prunes, and the like. When convalescence sets in, beef-tea and chicken broth should be given. Toast-water and oatmeal-water may be used as beverages which, with the diet, should be more cold than warm. To allay irritation and prevent pitting, the pustules should be painted with glycerine or starch.

Kali mur. is the principal remedy; it controls the formation of pustules.

Kali sulph. may be given to promote the formation of healthy skin and the falling off of the crusts.

SORE THROAT.

Treatment—Use a wet compress around the throat; gargle with water and take *Ferrum phos.*, a dose every half hour, if the throat is red, inflamed, painful; burning in throat. Useful for the sore throats of singers and those who use the voice much, Tendency to evening hoarseness.

Kali mur.—When tonsils swell. Ulcerated sore throat. Granular pharyngitis. Tough mucus in throat.

Natrum mur.—Sore throat of smokers and after nitrate of silver treatment. Throat feels constricted with stitches. Chronic sore throat with feeling of a plug or lump and great dryness.

Calcar. fiuor.—Relaxed sore throat, uvula too long tickling in throat. Hawking of mucus early in the morning. Burning in throat.

SPASMS.

Are usually met with in domestic practice in children, who are of a nervous organization and have been subjected to errors in diet. The first thing to do is to get rid of the offending cause, hence an injection or even vomiting may be resorted to A hot bath is always indicated. After these things have been attended to, give *Magnes phos.* dissolved in hot water every few minutes for a few doses. This may be followed by *Calcer. phos.*, especially if the *Mag. phos.* fails to give entire relief *Calc, phos.* is especially indicated in convulsions from teething without fever. Fits during development in childhood. In anemic, pale patient, cramps and convulsive movements of all kinds.

A dose three times a day beginning with the third, and after some time substituting the sixth and higher.

SPINAL IRRITATION.

Is shown by backache, painful spine, headache, impaired digestion. etc., frequently found in historical subjects. A course of the Tissue Remedies, together with attention to the general health, massage, salt water baths, will be of great benefit. The chies remedies are :

Natrum mur., especially when the patient is easily fatigued weakness from the slightest exertion, restless, Pain in back and head, spine very sensitive. Salty taste and repugnance to food ; vision becomes bim after reading ; skin dry and harsh, mouth dry ; feet heavy ; back feels broken ; bladder weak, dribbing of urine.

Silica.—Spinal irritation of children depending on warms. Nape of neck stiff—burning in back Patient very sensitive to every impression, feels better from warmth in general.

Kali Phos. may be give in alternation with either of these remedies as a general nerve food.

SUN STROKE

Remedis:

Nat. Mur. This is the chief remedy to regulate the distribution of moisture. To be given at frequent intervals.

Ferr. Phos. In alternation with Nat. Mur. for the inflammatory symptoms and to help respiration.

SYNOVITIS

Remedies:

Ferr. Phos. For the pains, stiffness and inflammation.

Nat. Sulph. To dispense the infiltration of fluid.

Silica For chronic Synovitis of the knee, with swelling and difficulty of movement.

Calc. Fluo. A useful tremedy in long-standing cases that are slow to respond the treatment.

TEETHING (Dentition).

There is no doubt that the teething process does predispose the child to various disturbances ; it renders it more sensitive and open to all sorts of impressions and morbid influences. There is more or less restlessness, sleeplessness, fever, bowel disturbance and skin irritation. Look to the general physical comfort of the child, warm clothing, sufficient but not too much bed clothing, regular bathing, good air, sunny room, daily exercise in the open air, if the weather permits, etc. Suitable food, of which mother's milk is the best of course, is of paramount importance. In the absence of mother's milk, cow's milk modified by the addition of barley-water is one of the best substitutes. When the teeth begin to appear, a crust of bread and broth may be given in addition, though milk should be the principal article of diet for the first four years. There is nothing more certain than the favouable influence of some of the Tissue Remedies in regulating this important time in the child's life.

Calcar. phas. If the teeth are rather late in erupting, it should be given to hosten development. It is the remedy for all troublesome ailments during dentition ; especially useful in flabby, emaciated children who are apt to have loose bowels and suffer from stomach troubles. No remedy has a greater or wider influence.

Calcar. fluor., which also greatly facilitates dentition ; indicated when there is vomiting and spasms, incessant crying, etc.

Magnes. phos. In convulsive cases, much twitching of muscles or complete spasms ; colic and loose bowels call for it. Should be given after every stool and during spasmodic symptoms every few minutes.

THRUSH (Ephthæ, Sore-mouth).

Treatment Liquid and cool food alone must be given. Keep the mouth scrupulously clean with a solution of Boracic acid or Ascepticon.

Kali mur. and *Natrum phosph.* are the remedies which may be given alternatively every hour.

TONGUE.

The appearence of the tongue gives very valuable indications for the use of the Tissue Remedies. Sometimes it alone, when very marked, may lead to the right remedy. The most marked appearances characteristic of each remedy are the following.

Kali mur.—Tongue swollen ; coating white, grayish shining.

Kali phosph.—Tongue excessively dry, brown, Edges red and sore,

Kali sulph.--Coating yellow, slimy with insipid, pappy taste.

Natrum mur.—Clean, moist tongue, sensation of a hair on tongue. *Feels* dry, but is not. Small bubbles of forthy saliva cover the sides and tips

Natrum phos.—Coating at the base moist, creamy or golden yellow.

Calcar. fluor.—Cracked appearance of tongue.

TONSILLITIS (Quinsy).

Remedies—Kali mur. is the principal remedy.

Calcar sulph.—If pus forms, it may then be alternated with the former.

Besides the remedies, ice is very gratefull Ice-cream will be found a good food.

TONSILS, ENGLARGED.

A very common affection of childhood, often interfering with breathing with mouth closed. Before resorting to cutting, which is so popular nowadays, a course of internal medication should be given a chance to cure radically. Frequently a few week's treatment will accomplish the result.

The principal remedy is *Calcar. phos.* Chronic swelling of the tonsils, causing pain on opening mouth, difficulty in swallowing and deafness, husky voice. Give the 2x trituration, one tablet four times a day for two weeks ; then substitute the 3x, and later the 6th given in the same way.

TOOTHACHE

Pain in one or more teeth, which varies extremely in degree, duration, and character, frequently extending to the face, ears, neck, and head, and often resulting from pregnancy, decayed teeth, extremes or sudden changes of tempreature, cold, rheumatism, indigestion, or from hot or cold, sweet or sour articles of food or drink, etc.

Remedies—Ferrum phosph., when there is heat and redness in the cheek and when pain is releved by cold drinks.

Natrum mur., when the pain is associated with profuse flow of tears or of saliva.

Magnes. phos., when the pains are relieved by the application of heat and warm drinks.

Silica, when the pains seem to be deep in the jaw.

Calcar. flour., when gum boil forms or other hard swelling.

Dose—A tablet of the selected remedy should be given every half of quarter of an hour. When improvement sets in, not so often.

TUMORS.

Nothing proves the efficiency of constitutional treatment by means of the Tissue Remedies more than the disappearance of growths and tumors after a course of this treatment. Not all yield ; probably none in the latter stages of their development, but many in the earlier stages ; and it is certain that surgical measures should not be decided upon until a few months' treatment has been tried.

Kali phos. has been found of much use in cancer, for the pain, offensive discharge and debility.

Kali sulph., in epithelioma, cancer on the skin near a mucous lining with discharge of thin, mattery secretion.

Calcar. phos. Cysts of all sorts require this remedy. Goitre, weeping sinew, housemaids' knee, etc., all yield to this drug.

Calc. fluor.—Hard tumors. Knots, kernels, hardend glands in the breast. Indurated lumps.

Silica.—Enlarged glands ; swellings lumps that are hard but threaten to suppurate,

TYPHOID FEVER

Remedies : *Calc. phos.* 3x, 6x—After typhoid to regain health ; It is a great restorative.

Ferr. phos. 3x, 6x—First stage, pain, haemorrhage of bright red blood.

Kali mur. 3x, 6x—The most useful remedy. Grey-white coating on the tongue. Stools loose, light yellow. Haemorrhage of dark clotted blood.

Kali phos. 6x, 12x—Malignant symptoms ; offensive stools ; great weakness and prostration. Delirium ; weak and irregular pulse ; yellow-white coating on the tongue.

ULCERS.

Here, too, the administration of internal remedies does more than all local measures ever accomplished. These are not to be neglected but healthy action is greatly furthered by the concomitant use of the Tissue Remedies.

Silica.—Always indicated in suppurative processes, glandular swellings with suppuration. Ulcers of the lower limbs ; spongy, easily bleeding ulcers ; sluggish ulcers, in hard worked and ill-fed persons. Ulceration following abrasion of the skin over the shin-bone.

URINARY TROUBLES.

Ferrum phos.—One of the best remedies for wetting oi the bed in chlidren and incontinence of urine when every cough causes the urine to spurt. Inflammation of the bladder; irresistible urging to urinate, aggravated by standing, with smarting and pain.

Kali phos.—wetting of the bed in older children. Incontinence in old people; scalding, bloody urine; itching of urethra.

Magnes. phos.—Spasmodic retention of urine. Gravel.

Natrum phos.—Chief remedy in catarrh of the bladder. Much mucus in urine; frequent urination; diabetes.

Natrum sulph.—Sandy deposit, gravel, brick-dust sediment. Especially useful in gouty patients. This remedy is advantageously followed by.

Calcur. phos.—Tendency to stone in the bladder; flocculent sediment.

Nutrum mur.—Cutting in urethra, and after urinating; much and frequent urine; involuntary, after coughing, when walking, etc., etc.

VACCINATION.

Should any ill effects show themselves after vaccination, *Kali mur.* and *Silica* will neutralize them; a dose of one in the morning and the other at night.

VARICOSE VEINS.

Enlarged veins, more especially in the legs, and occurring frequently during pregnancy. They are discolored, knotty, and sometimes become very painful, and may burst, if neglected.

Ferrum phos. is a powerful vein remedy. Varicose veins in young persons; throbbing in the parts.

Calcar. fluor. is the chief remedy for all forms of varicose veins. Sharp, piercing pains, burning, soreness, even ulceration of the veins.

VERTIGO.

Is a symptom of various diseased conditions: may be caused by gastric disorders as well as disturbed of the circulation.

Remedies—If due to congestion of the brain, shown by hot head, full pulse, etc , give *Ferrum phosph* , a dose every two hours. If due to anemic condition, give *Calcar. phos.*, a dose there times a day. If due to gastric disorders, consult the remedies there indicated.

Kali phos. in the aged; vertigo worse rising or looking up; nervous causes ; run-down states of the system.

Natrum sulph., with biliousness and bitter taste ; excess of bile.

VOICE, LOSS OF.

Usually from cold or over use of voice. Rest, warm drinks, and *Ferrum phos*, every hour, usually soon restore the voice.

VOMITING.

If bilious, see under "Bilious Attacks."

This is a frequent symptom in children from errors in diet or at the beginning of acute diseases, notably brain troubles in adults it indicates diseases of the stomach of kidneys, most commonly an excess of bile, so-called biliousness.

In order to treat it successfully, the whole patient must be taken into consideration and the underlying complaint treated, but the symptom is very marked in the following remedies.

Silica—Child vomits as soon as it nurses. Morning vomiting with chilliness.

Ferrum phos.—Vomiting of food with sour fluids, soon after eating ; vomiting of blood, bright red.

Kali mur. Vomiting of thick, white phlegm.

Natrum mur.—Vomiting of sour fluid, not food; curdled masses ; dark substance, like coffee-grounds; of watery, stringy transparent mucus.

Natrum phos.—Vomiting of sour fluid curdy masses with yellow coating of tongue.

Natrum sulph.—Bilious vomiting with bitter taste. Morning sickness, constant nausea.

Calcer phos.—Vomiting after cold water and ice-cream. Infant vomits often and easily and want to nurse all the time.

Vomiting with teething troubles.

WHOOPING COUGH.

Symptoms—In the catarrhal stage are those of an ordinary cold—sneezing, watery discharge from the nose, watery eyes, hoarseness, dry cough, headache, oppression at the chest, feverish nights. etc., lasting for two or three weeks.

In the convulsive or whooping stage there are violent paroxysms of cough of a convulsive and suffocative character, and distinguished by a peculiar whoop. The face and neck are sometimes swollen and livid, the eyes protruded and full of tears. The duration of the paroxysms varies from one to five minutes, at the termination of which there is often vomiting or expectoration of food or ropy mucus. This stage lasts from five to six weeks.

Treatment—The diet must be nourishing and the strength of the patient well kept up. Plenty of fresh air and regular exercise should be enjoined. Linseed tea, or gum-arabic water will be found useful to allay the irritability of the throat. All sources of irritation and excitement should be excluded from the invalid.

Magnes. phos. is the principal remedy. It should be given steadily, and will soon greatly modify the disease.

Calcer. phos. may de needed in weakly constitutions, or in teething children, and in obstinate cases with emaciation.

WORMS, THERAD.

Treatment—Look to the diet ; avoid too much starchy and amylacious food, mushes etc. It may be necessary to give an occasional injection of salt and water, one teaspoonful to a quart of water, and afterwards apply a little vaseline to the rectum. Keep the parts immaculately clean.

Natrum phos. is the principal remedy for all kinds of worms—round, long or thread worms. There may be pain in the bowels, restless sleep, picking at nose, acidity, itching of rectum, grinding of teeth, etc., all symptoms more or less present with this trouble. This remedy probably acts by destroying the excess of lactic acid, which seems to be necessary for the life of these worms Give one tablet of the third potency night and morning.

WOUNS, SPRAINS AND STRAINS.

Remedies :—

Ferrum phos. This is the first remedy for sprains, bruises, cuts, wounds, etc., It alleviates pain and congestion and should be applied externally wherever possible.

Kali mur. For the swelling in alternation with *Ferr. phos.*

Calc. sulph. Bruises, cuts, wounds, etc. when neglected and suppurating.

Calc. Fluo. Bruises affecting the bones.

Silica. Neglected wounds with festering. Discharges of thickyellow pus.

Nat. sulph. For the shock and after-effects.

Calc. phos. For fracture of bones to help the fracture to mend. This should be given in all cases where there is injury or brittleness of the bones.

WRITER'S CRAMP.

The treatment consist in rest largely, massage and the administration of *Natrum phos*. and *Magnes*. A dose of one in the morning and the other a night for some weeks. If necessary, these may be followed by *Calcar., phos.*, especially where there is cramplike pain in figers and wrists.

———

Materia Medica

CALCAREA FLUORICA (Fluoride of Lime).

This salt is found in the surface of the bones and in the enamel of the teeth ; also in the elastic fibres and skin. A disturbance of the equilibrium of the molecules of this salt, according to the theory of Biochemistry, causes a relaxed condition and a dilatation, interfering with absorption and hence favoring hardening and swelling of the tissues. Enlarged veins, piles, swollen and hardened glands, tumors, uterine displacements, are conditions resulting from such a cause.

Head—Lumps on head ; hard swellings ; nasal troubles : stuffy cold ; bad odor with thick, lumpy discharge, which is hard to detach, going back into throat.

Mouth and Throat—Gumboil with hard swelling on the jaw ; cold sores ; throat troubles, tickling from enlarged soft palate.

Stomach and Bowels—Hiccough and vomiting ; constipation and piles, swollen and hard ; bleeding piles ; itching of rectum ; internal piles, with backache ; displacement of the womb, indicated by dragging pains, falling of womb ; profuse menstruation.

Respiratory Organs—The chief remedy in croup ; dry, hoarse cough ; tickling and cough, with lumps of thick mucus.

Extremities and Skin—Enlarged veins ; chief remedy for varicose veins anywhere ; blood tumors ; gouty enlargements : cracking in joints ; weeping sinew ; inflammation of knee-joint hardened ; glands, knots and kernels, and tumors anywhere.

Corresponding Homeopothic Remedies—Fluoric acid, Aurum and Silica.

For hard swellings—Baryta jod., Calcar. jod,

For offensive catarrh—Aurum and Kali bich.

CALCAREA PHOSPHORICA (Phosphate of Lime).

This salt gives solidity to the bones. It is absolutely exssention to the proper growth and nutrition of the body and supplies the first basis for the new tissues. An insufficient supply of Calcarea phos. results in defective nutrition, imperfect growt hand decay. It is of greatest importance during dentition, in young, rapidly growing children, at puberty, in old age and especially after acute diseases, drains on the system and in inherited weakness and disease tendencies, especially scrofulous and tuberculous manifestations.

Head—Peevish and fretful state ; impaired memory ; vertigo, cold feeling in head ; headache, at puberty ; in infants, bones of head do not close ; scalp sore, itches, feels cold.

Eyes and Ears—Scrofulous inflammation of eyes with spots on cornea ; eye-troubles in school children and at the time of puberty ; cannot use eyes by gas light ; twitching of lids ; bon:r around ear ache ; ear feels cold.

Face—Pimples ; complexion sallow, greasy ; face-ache.

Mouth and Throat—Bad taste ; teeth develop slowly; difficult teething ; glands swollen ; chronic enlargements of tonsils ; relaxed sore throat ; sore throat with pain on swallowing ; constant hawking.

Stomach—Flatulence and heartburn ; infant wants to nurse all the time ; pains after eating ; craving for salted and smoked meat.

Abdomen—Stool is watery, offensive, noisy ; summer complaints ; pain in rectum ; fistula.

Urinary and Sexual—Wetting of the bed ; incontinence in old people ; diabetes ; gravel ; utrine displacements, with rheumatic pains ; menses too early and too profuse. After prolonged nursing, leucorrhea, etc., it acts as a constitutional tonic.

Respiratory—Soreness of chest ; cough of consumptives ; palpitation.

Extermities—Rheumatism ; numb, cold limbs ; sore, aching, worse any change of weather ; languor, rembling and twitching ; anemia and chlorosis ; rickets ; flabby, emaciated, sickly, ailing, backward children; polypi; irregularity in development; lumbago, after the use of Ferrum phos; housemaids knee; bow-legs in children and swelling of the joints.

Corresponding Homeopathic Remedies—China, Ruta and Symphytum.

As a remedy for the aged, Baryta is often more valuable.

In children, Calcar. carb. is to be preferred, when they are fair, plump, sweat much, with cold, damp feet much of the time.

CALCAREA SULPHURICA (Gypsum)

This salt is contained in the connective tissue and it stands in close relation to suppurations. It cures at that stage, when suppuration continues too long. The presence of pus with a vent is the general indication.

Head—Scald head of children; pimples and pustubes on face; cold in head with thick discharge; edges of nostrils sore.

Respiratory—Cough with hestic fever; obstinate hoarseness; bronchitis; consumption; catarrh with thick, lumpy, pus-like secretions; cough with herpetic eruptions.

Extremities; Backache; burning itching of soles; herpetic eruptions all over; boils . carbuncles : chilblains; abscesses; to shorten the suppurative process; felons, ulecrs, with excessive granulations.

Corresponding Homeopathic Remedies—Hepar and Silica.

Calcer. sulph. resembles Hepar, but act deeper and more intensely, and is often useful after Hepar has ceased to act. Silica is preferable in glands that suppurate.

FERRUM PHOSPHORICUM (Phosphate of Iron).

Iron is found in the red blood corpuscles most abundantly, but is contained also in every cell. A disturbance of the equilibrium of the iron molecules in the muscular fibres causes a relaxed condition, favoring congestion and hemorrhage. Iron restores the tone, equalizes the circulation, and abates the fever. All ailments of a congestive nature, especially in children who are dull and listless, failing appetite, lose weight, etc.

Head and face—Rush of blood to head ; throbbing headcaches ; head sore to touch, with eyes bloodshot, red, inflamed ; florid complexion ; hot, red face ; face-ache, with flushed face, cheek sore and hot ; cold applications are grateful ; gums hot ; teething troubles, with feverishness.

Nose and Ears—First stage of all colds ; bleeding from nose ; noises in ears, earache ; deafness.

Throat—Throat dry, red, inflamed, painful; first stage of diptheria and ulcerated throat.

Gastric symptoms—Thirst ; vomiting of food and blood ; undigested stools ; hemorrhoids and dysentery.

Urinary symptoms, etc.—Wetting of the bed ; frequent urination ; menses too early, and frequent, and profuse ; menstrual colic.

Respiratory symptoms—First remedy for colds on the chest, especially in children. Painful cough with fever ; soreness of chest ; cough with emission of urine ; cough with bloody expectoration ; bronchitis, pleurisy and pneumonia in the first stage ; croup ; loss of voice ; hoarseness ; huskiness after talking or singing ; whooping cough with vomiting; palpitation.

Back and Extremities—Stiff neck ; lumbago ; rheumatic pains anywhere, that are worse moving and better from warmth ; acute articular rheumatism.

Corresponding Homeopathic Remedies—Aconite and Gelsemium,

Aconite has more restless, ness tossing about and greater fever.

Gelsem., more drowsiness and languor.

In anemic conditions, China and Calcar. phos.

In respiratory troubles, Bryonia and Tartar emetic follow often.

KALI MURIATICUM (Chloride of Potash).

This salt is found in the blood, nerve cells and muscles. It stands in a chemical relation to fibrin and corresponds to the second stage of all inflammations. Croupous and diphtheritic membranes, lymphatic enlargements, discharges and expectorations of thick, whitish matter. The principal indications for the drug are such discharges and white, greyish coating of the tongue. The efficacy of this remedy is demonstrated in chronic catarrhal conditions, croup, diphtheria, dysentery, pneumonia. In alternation with Ferr. phos. in coughs, deafness from from catarrh of the Eustachian tubes, skin eruptions with small vesicles containing yellowish secretions, ulcerations with swellings and white exudations ; in leucorrhea with characteristic discharges, etc. Symptoms in general are worse from motion ; the gastric and abodominal being worse after taking pastry, rich and fatty foods.

Head symptoms—Sick headache ; dandruff and eruptions on scalp ; chronic discharge from ears ; deafness and earache; noises in ears ; stuffy colds ; thrush, canker and rawness of mouth ; tongue coated grayish, white and slimy.

Throat—It is useful most cases of diphtheria and specific for diphtheritic sore throat ; pharyngitis, tonsilitis ; chronic sore throat with deafness.

Gastric Symptoms—Dyspepsia with a whitish gray tongue after rich food ; vomiting of white mucus; jaundice, sluggish action of liver ; constipation with furred tongue ; abdomen tender ; diarrhea after fatty food ; piles, especially bleeding, dysentery.

Urinary and Sexual Organs—Inflammation of bladder ; dark colored urine, with sandy deposits ; Urethritis, menses too late, leucorrhea, thick and bland ; ulceration of womb ; morning sickness, and inflammation of the breast.

Respiratory Organs—Loss of voice ; asthma, cough, with thick, whitish expectoration, croup, pleurisy and pnenmonia, after Ferrum phos.

Back and Extremities—Rheumatism with swelling around joints ; rheumatic pains felt only during motion, or at night in bed ; epilepsy.

Skin—Abscesses, boils, carbuncles, acne, eczema, burns, cold sores, pimples, pustuls, warts, etc., all require a course of Kali mur., chief remedy in glandular swellings, old spasmodic conditions.

Corresponding Homeopathic Remedies—Bryonia Merrcurius and Sulphur. Like Sulphur, it is a deep acting remedy with eradlcating tendencies, useful as an inter-current medicine in the treatment of chronic diseases.

KALI PHOSPHORICUM (Phosphate of Potash)

This salt is a constituent of all animal fluids and tissue, notably of the brain, nerves, muscles and blood. It si an antiseptic and hinders the decay of tissues. Nervous conditions known as neurasthenic, is the field in which this salt has become pre-eminent. The results of a want of nerve power, as prostration, exertion, loss of mental vigor, depression, brain-feg, softening of the brain, and when there is rapid decomposition of the blood. It is curative in septic hemorrhages, scorbutic gangrene, stomatitis, offensive carrion-like diarrhea or dysentery, adynamic or typhoid conditions, incontinence of urine, urticaria, predisposition to epistaxis in children, dizziness and vertigo from nervous exhaustion; tongue coated as if spread with dark liquid mustard. Many symptoms are aggravated by noise; by rising from a sitting position; by exertion, physical and mental; pains worse in cold air; ameliorated by gentle motion, eating, excitement, anything in fact that will relieve the mind and aid in restoring the lacking nerve force. Typhoid and gastric fever, malignant conditions.

Head Symptoms—Nervous dread, anxiety and fear; brain-fag; depressed spirits; general irritability; impaired memory; dulness, want of energy, hysteria, nervousness and weakness; headaches of students and those worn out; very sensitive to noise and other impressions; confused feeling—here follow with Calc. fluor., second potency.

Gastric—Tongue dry; feels as if it would cleave to roof of mouth; coated dark brown; edges sore and red; bleeding of gums; hungry feeling; all gone sensation; constant pain in pit of stomach; flatulence; diarrhea, rectum sore; bowel prolapsed; stools dark brown, bloody, offensive.

Back and Extremities—Paralytic conditions; burning of feet, fidgety feeling, numbness and weakness; neuralgic pains anywhere with depression; weakness, sciatica; cold aggravates all pains.

Respiratory Organs—Short breath, hoarseness, faintness; intermittent and irregular pulse, palpition.

Urinary Organs—In wetting of the bed of children, this remedy is often effective when other remedies fail. Frequent urination in old people ; diabetes with nervous weakness ; Bright's disease. Menses premature and profuse, black and offensive ; dull headache with menses, very tired and sleepy, legs ache ; pain in ovaries and across lower part of back ; yellow leucorrhoea.

Corresponding Homoeopathic Remedies—Rhus and Phosphorus, Pulsatilla and Ignatia. The nearest analogue is Rhus, for the symptoms depending on blood changes while Phosphorus is more like it in the nervous diseases. As a nerve sedative, Kali phos. corresponds with Ignatia and Coffea. In menstrual headaches Gelsemium, Pulsatilla and Cimicifuga.

KALI SULPHURICUM (Sulphate of Potash).

The skin and mucous membrane are largely under the influence of this salt. It is especially called for in the late stages of all inflammations. In profuse desquamation. In all conditions accompanied by a yellow mucous discharge or caused by suppression of eruptions or discharge. When the patient is worse towards evening and better in the open air.

Head—Dizziness and headache, worse in warm room and in the evening ; dandruff and scald head ; eruptions on scalp ; colds, with yellow slimy matter ; old catarrhs, nose obstructed, lost smell ; offensive discharge.

Gastric Symptoms—Burning thirst ; catarrh of stomach with yellow, slimy coated tongue ; pressure as of a load in stomach ; dread of hot drinks ; yellow, slimy diarrhea, with colic ; habitual constipation.

Urinary and Sexual—Slimy, yellow or greenish discharge from urethra or from vagina.

Respiratory Organs—Bronchial asthma and catarrh, worse in warm season ; cough worse in the evening ; great rattling in the chest ; rattling of mucus with cough ; suffocative feeling in hot atmosphere ; desire for cool air.

Extremities—Rheumatic pains in back and extremities, shifting, wandering, settling in one place, then in another.

Skin—Inactive skin ; chafing of skin ; scaly tetters ; ivy-poison ; nettle rash ; burning, itching eruptions ; diseased nails; erysipelas ; and eczema and cancerous growth ; polypi.

Corresponding Homoeopatic Remedies—Pulsatilla is the nearest analogue. Kali sulph. often follows very advantageously Kali mur. and Pulsatilla.

MAGNESIA PHOSPHORICA (Phosphate of Magnesia).

This salt is a constituent of muscles and nerves. It causes contraction in muscular fibres and hence its use in cramps, convulsions and other nervous disturbances. Pains anywhere that are relieved by warmth and pressure. It is the great antispasmodic remedy. It acts best when given in hot water.

Head—Pain in head always relieved by warm application; neuralgia with chilliness after mental labor ; neuralgia around eyes, worse on right side ; earache worse from cold air. or caused by washing in cold water ; face-ache, worse touch, cold wind, washing, better by application of heat ; convulsive twitching of facial muscles or eyelids ; toothache ; complaints of teething children, especially spasmodic symptoms.

Gastric Symptoms—Hiccough, heartburn, gastralgia, flatulent dyspepsia ; flatulent colic relieved by warmth and pressure ; abdomen bloated, watery diarrohea with cramps ; constipation of infants, with spasmodic pain at every attempt at stool with much gas.

Female Symptoms—Menstrual colic ; pain precedes flow : intermittent ; ovarian neuralgia ; membranous discharge with menses ; menses too early, dark, fibrous.

Respiratory Organs—Whooping cough, best remedy ; any spasmodic cough, worse at night and on lying down ; oppression of chest ; constriction of chest and throat ; angina pectoris ; nervous palpitation.

Back and Extremities—Neuralgic pains ; intercostal neuralgia ; tingling sensations ; feet very tender ; cramps in calves ; neuralgia in limbs with musular contractions ; languid and exhausted feeling ; chorea ; bad effects from stimulants.

Corresponding Homoeopathic Remedies—The most striking resemblance of its action is to Colocynthis which may be used with it in colic and neuralgic affections. In spasmodic symptoms, Belladonna is similar. In female complaints, it is very similar to Pulsatilla and Cimicifuga.

NATRUM MURIATICUM (Chloride of Sodium or Common Salt).

This is a constituent of every liquid and solid of the body. It regulates the degree of moisture within the cells. Wherever we find a hypersecretion of the watery elements of the body, with simultaneous want of activity in some other portion of the mucous membranes, you will find Natrum mur. the remedy. It acts upon the lymphatic system, the blood, liver, spleen, and upon the mucous lining of the alimentary canal. Natrum mur. is indicated in headache, toothache, face-ache, stomachache, etc., where there is either salivation or hyper-secretion of tears, or vomiting of water and mucus; also catarrhal affections of mucous membranes, with secretion of transparent, watery, frothy mucus ; also small watery blisters, breaking and leaving a thin crust ; diarrohea, transparent, glossy, slimy stools ; coujuctivitis with discharge of tears and clear mucus ; tongue clear, slimy, small bubbles of frothy saliva on sides ; leucorrhea, watery, smarting or clear, starch-like discharge, etc. etc.

Head—Very depressed in spirit, hypochondriacal mood with constipation and brain-fag ; hammering headache worse in morning ; sick. headache with constipation ; muscles of neck feel weak itching eruption on margin of hair at the nape of neck ; inflamed eyelids ; neuralgia around eyes ; impaired vision ; old nasal catarrh ; loss of smell and taste ; sallow complexion ; cold sores on lips.

Gastric Symptoms—Waterbrash ; ravenous hunger, violent thirst ; aversion to bread ; heartburn ; offensive breath ; constipatian, smarting after stool ; piles and fissures.

Urinary—Frequent urination ; catarrh of bladder ; burning and soreness in vagina after urinating ; very melancholy about the time of menses ; prolapse and smarting leucorrhea.

Back and Extremities—Backache better by lying on something hard; pain in hip ; weakness of legs ; cracking of joints.

Corresponding Homoeopathic Remedies—Sepia and Sulphur—These frequently are of service after Natrum mur. For the ill-effects of excessive use of salt in food, give Phosphorus 30,

NATRUM PHOSPHORICUM (Phosphate of soda).

This salt is found in the blood, muscles and nerve cells and in the inter-cellular fluids. Through its presence, conditions arising from excess of lactic acid are prevented. It serves to emulsify fatty acids and is therefore a remedy for all dyspeptic conditions traceable to fats. This is the remedy in all cases where there is an excess of acidity. Acts also upon the bowels, glands, lungs and abdominal organs. It cures sour belchings and rising of fluids ; sour vomiting ; greenish, sour-smelling diarrhea, colic, spasms, fever from acidity of the stomach in children ; ague with characteristic coating of tongue ; eyes discharging a yellow creamy matter ; gastric derangements with acidity and flatulence ; indigestion, intestinal worms, etc. A characteristic indication is a moist, thick, golden-yellow coating on the tongue and palate.

Head—Giddiness, with gastric derangements ; sick headaches with sour vomiting.

Gastric—Yellow, creamy coating at the back part of roof of mouth and on tongue ; grinding of teeth. Acidity, sour risings ; pain after food ; nausea and vomiting ; flatulence, colic with acidity ; stomach-ache from presence of worms ; itching of rectum.

Respiratory—A useful intercurrent remedy in catarrhal troubles associated with acidity. Pain in chest from pressure and breathing ; consumption ; pulpitation, pulse felt in different parts of body.

Back and Extremities—Weak feeling ; legs give way while walking ; pain in knees and ankles ; aching wrists.

Corresponding Homeopathic Remedies—Calcar. carb. and Rheum, especially for children where there is much acid condition of stomach and bowels.

NATRUM SULPHURICUM (Glauber's Salt).

This salt does not appear in the cells, only in the intercellular fluids. It aids and regulates the excretion of superfluous water. Gastric bilious conditions, dropsy, liver diseases, results of living in damp, low dwellings or regions, uric acid diathesis, all are benefited by this remedy. The chief characteristic symptom is the appearance of the tongue—durty, greenish brown.

Head—Sick headache with bilious diarrohea ; violent pain at base of brain ; mental troubles arising from injuries to the head.

Gastric—Bitter taste ; mouth full of slime, thick and tenacious, must hawk it up ; tongue coated dirty, brownish, vomiting of bile ; flatulent colic ; diarrhea, stools dark, bilious, worse in morning, particularly after wet weather ; great size of the fecal mass ; aching in region of liver.

Urinary—Chief remedy in diabetes ; sandy deposit in urine like brick-dust in the water.

Respiratory—Asthma, worse in damp weather, cough with thick, ropy expectoration ; bronchial catarrh ; cough worse in early morning ; difficult breathing ; asthma in children from suppression of skin troubles.

Back and Extremities—Soreness up and down spine and back ; drawing back of neck ; pain under nails ; sciatica ; gout ; twitching during sleep ; intermittent fever in all its stages ; dropsy.

Corresponding Homoeopathic Remedies—Thuja and Sulphur—In the cough, Bryonia, but this is indicated rather earlier in chest affections than Natrum sulph., and hence the latter often follows it advantageously.

SILICA (Pure Quartz).

This salt, though very abundantly found in the vegetable kingdom, is found only in the connective tissue to any extent. It acts prominently upon the bones, glands, skin, and is especially suited to the imperfectly nourished constitutions. It is the remedy for ailments attended with pus-formation. It ripens abscesses and promotes suppuration. Especially indicated in sensitive patients, who are always chilly.

Head—Oversensitive, irritable ; vertigo ; headache coming up from nape of neck, worse on right side, worse from noise, exertion, light, study ; better from warmth ; styes.

Gastric—Child vomits as soon as it nurses ; chronic dyspepsia ; disgust for meat and warm food ; very hungry; large abdomen ; paralytic condition of bowels ; patient is cold all the time ; menses are associated with icy coldness and constipation, and fetid foot-sweat.

Respiratory—Cough of sickly children, with night-sweats hoarseness ; tickling cough ; cough and sore throat, with expectoration of little granules ; smelling badly ; deep-seated pain in chest ; much pus-like expectoration ; chronic heart disease.

Back and Extermities—Spinal irritation ; soreness between shoulders ; hip-joint disease ; whitlow, felon ; nails crippled and brittle ; habitual fetid perspiration of the feet or axillæ ; ingrowing toe-nails ; pains in feet ; weak ankles ; skin heals with difficulty, and suppurates easily ; skin very sensitive ; all sorts of eruptions and ulcerations ; enlarged suppurating glands ; patient feels better in warm room, and by heat generally.

Corresponding Homoeopathic Remedies—Mercurius and Pulsatilla, Picric acid. In suppuration, Calcar. sulph. is better adapted to checking it and healing, promoting healthy granulation. It follows Silica. Silica often follows very advantageously, Pulsatilla and Calcarea.

Repertory

Mental States.

Ambitionless, *Natr. phas.*
Angry, *Nat. mur.*
Apprehensive, *Kali phos.*
Anxiety, *Calc. phos.*, *Kali phos.*
Brain fag, *Kali. phos.*, *Silica.*
Changeable mood, *Calc. sulph.*
Confused feeling, *Calc. fluor.*
Crying Mood, *Kali phos.*
Depressed mood, *Natr. mur.*
Despairs getting well, *Natr. sulph.*
Despondency, *Kali phos.*
Difficult thought, *Silica,*
Dread, nervous, *Kali phos.*
Fear of falling, *Kali sulph.*
Fear of financial ruin, *Calc. fluor.*
Forgetful, *Calc. phos.*
Fretful, *Kali phos.*
Hallucinations, *Kali phos.*, *Natr. phos.*
Indifference *Ferrum phos.*
Indecision, *Calc. fluor.*
Insanity, *Ferr. phos.*, . *Kali phos.*
Melancholia, *Kali phos.*, *Natr. sulph.*
Night terrors, *Kali phos.*
Over-sensitive, *Silica Kali. phos.*
Passionate outbursts, *Nat. mur.*
Sadness, *Nat. mur.*
Screaming, *Kali phos.*
Sighing, *Nat. mur.*
Slow comprehension, *Calc. phos.*
Suicidal tendency, *Nat sulph.*
Whining, *Kali phos.*

Head

Bald spots, *Kali sulph.*
Brain-fag, *Silica. Kali phos.*
Burning on top, *Nat. sulp.*
Cold feeling, *Calc. phos.*
Congestive headache, *Ferr. phos.*
Dandruff, *Kali sulph.*, *Nat. mur.*
Effects of injuries to, *Nat. sulph.*
Falling out of hair, *Kali sulph.*
Fontanelles unclosed, *Calc. phos.*
Headache, congestive, *Ferr. phos.*
Headache, menstrul, *Nat. mur.*
" sick, *Nat sulph.*
Lumps on scalp, *Silica.*
Soreness to touch, *Ferr. phos.*
Sunstroke, *Nat mur.*
Sweat on head, *Calc. phos.*, *Silica.*

Throbbing, *Ferr phos*
Vertigo, old age, *Calc. phos.*
" with bile, *Nat. sulph.*
Yellow crusts on scald. *Calc. sulph.*

Eyes

Agglutination of lids, *Nat. phos.*
Asthenopia, *Nat. mur.*
Black spots before, *Kali phos.*
Blisters on, *Nat. mur,*
Blood shot, *Nat. phos.*
Burning of lids, *Nat. sulph.*
Conjunctivitis, *Ferr. phos., Nat. phos.*
Dull vision, *Nat. phos.*
Eye-ball, sore, *Ferr. phos.*
Eyelids, granular, *Nat. mur.*
Pupils contracted, *Magnes. phos.*
Redness, *Ferr. phos., Nat. mur*
Styes *Silica.*

Ears

Aching around, *Calc. phos*
Buzzing in, *Kali. phos.*
Catarrh, *Kali. mur.*
Deafness. *Ferr. phos., Kali. mur.*
Discharge from, *Kali phos., Silica.*
Earache, *Ferr .phos., Magnes. phos.*
Noises in, *Ferr. phos. Kali phos.*
Ringing, as of bells, *Nat. sulph.*

Nose

Bleeding, *Ferr. phos.*
Catarrh, *Kali mur.*
" old, chronic, *Nat. mur., Silica.*
Colds, *Ferr. phos.*
" stuffy ; *Kali sluph., Nat. mur.*
Crusts, *Kali mur., Silica.*
Discharge, acrid, *Silica.*
" clear, *Nat mur.*
" fetid, *Kali phos.*
" greenish, *Kali sulph.*
" thick. *Calc. fluor., Kali sulph.*
" yellow, *Nat. phos.*
Dry coryza *calc. fluor. Kali mur.*
Hay-fever, *Nat. mur., Slica.*
Influenza, *Nat. sulph.*
Loss of smell, *Nat. mur.*
Nostrils sore, *Calc. phos.,*
Odor. offensive, *Kali. phos., Calc. fluor.*
Pimples on, *Nat. mur.*
Posterior nares, dry, *Nat mur.*
" hawking form, *Kali, phos.*
Predisposition to take cold, *Calc. phos.*
Running colds, *Nat. mur.*
Sneezing, *Kali phos., Silica.*

Face

Acne, *Calc. sulph., Kali mur.*
Blotched, *Nat. phos.*
Cold sores, *Nat. mur., Calc. flour.*
Eruptions, *Calc. sulph., Kali sulph.*
Face-ache, *Magnes. phos., Ferr. phos.*
Greasy, *Calc phos.*
Hot, *Ferr. phos.*
Jaundiced, *Nat. sulph.*
Pale, *Nat. mur., Clac. phos.*

Red, *Ferr. phos.*
Sallow, *Nat. sulph.*
Yellowish, *Nat. sulph.*

Mouth

Aphthæ, *Kali mur.*
Breath, offensive, *Kali phos., Nat. mur.*
Cold-sores, *Nat. mur., Calc. fluor.*
Drooling, *Nat. mur.*
Gumboil, *Kali. mur.*
Gums, spongy, *Kali phos.*
Lips, crack, *Nat. mur.*
Salivation, *Nat. mur., Kali phos.*
Twitching, *Magnes. phos.*
Ulcer in *Kali, mur.*

Tongue and Taste

Acrid taste, *Nat. phos.*
Bitter taste, *Nat. sulph.*
Blisters on tongue, *Nat. mur.*
Brown tongue, *Kali phos., Nat. sulph.*
Cracked tongue, *Calc. fluor.*
Creamy tongue, *Nat. phos.*
Dry tongue, *Kali phos.*
Flabby tongue, *Calc. sulph.*
Frothy tongue *Nat. mur.*
Loss of taste. *Nat. mur.*
Mapped tongue. *Nat. mur.*
Numb tongue, *Calc. phos.*
Slimy tongue, *Kali sulph.*
Sour taste, *Calc. sulph.*
Ulcers on tongue, *Silica, Kali mur.*

Teeth and Gums.

Complaints during teething, *Calc. phos.*
Convulsions during, teething *Mag. phos.*
Decay of teeth, *Calc. phos.*
Dental fistula, *Silica.*
Drooling *Nat. mur.*
Enamel, deficient, *Calc. fluor.*
Grinding of teeth, *Nat. phos.*
Gumboil, *Kali. mur.*
" hard, swollen, *Calc. flour.*
" suppurating, *Calc. sulph.*
Gums, bleed easily, *Nat. mur.*
" inflamed *Calc. phos.*
" sensitive, *Nat. mur.*
Looseness of teeth, *Calc. Fluor.*

Throat

Burning, *Ferr. phos.*
Choking sensation, *Magnes. phos.*
Chronic sore. *Nat. mur. Kali mur.*
Clergyman's *Calc. phos.*
Constriction *Magnes. phos.*
Croup and Diphtheria, *Ferr. phos, Kali mur.*
Dryness, *Nat. mur.*
Dry throat, *Ferr. phos.*
Feeling of lump, *Nat. sulph.*
Follicular pharyngitis, *Kali. mur.* Nat. *mur.*
Glands, swollen *Kali mur.*
" suppurating, *Silica.*
Goitre, *Calc. fluor.*
Mumps, *Kali mur. Nat. mur.*
Posterior nares dropping, *Nat. phos.*
Relaxed sore throat, *Calc. phos.*
" uvula, *Nat. mur.*

Ulcerated sore throat, *Kali mur.*
Uvula, elongated, *Nat. mur.*

Gastric Symptoms.

Acids, sensitive to, *Magnes. phos.*
Acidity, Nat. *phos.*
Appetite, loss of, Kali *mur.*, *Calc. phos.*
Aversion to bread, Nat. *mur.*
" " hot drinks, *Kali suplh.*
" " meat, *Ferr. phos.*, *Silica*,
" " milk, *Ferr. phos.*
" " warm food, *Silica.*
Biliousness, *Nat. sulph.*
Burning in stomach, *Kali sulph.*
Desire for bacon, *Calc. phos.*
" " bitter things, *Nat. mur.*
" " claret, *Calc. sulph.*
" " fruits, *Calc. sulph.*
" " ham, *Calc. phos.*
" " salted food, *Calc. phos.*
" " stimulants, *Ferr. phos.*
" " sugar *Magnes. phos.*
Empty, gone feeling, *Kali Phos.*
Eructations, bitter, *Kali phos.*
" " burning, *Magnes. phos.*
" " gaseous, *Kali phos.*, *Calc. phos.*
" " greasy, *Ferr. phos.*
" " sour, *Nat. phos.*
Excessive hunger, *Silica.*
Faintness at stomach, *Kali sulph.*
Flatulence, *Calc. phos.*
" " with acidity, *Nat. phos. Calc. phos.*
Flatulence palpitation *Nat phos.*
" " sluggish liver, *Nat. sulph.*
Gastralgia, *Magnes. phos.*
Gastritis, *Ferr. phos.*
Heartburn, *Nat. mur. Silica.*
Hiccough, *Magne. phos. Calc. flour.*
Hunger, excessive, *Silca. Kali phos.*
Nausea, *Kali sulph. Ferr. phos.*
Nausea and vertigo, *Calc. sulph.*
Nausea and vomiting, *Magnes. phos.*
Pain after food. *Nat. phos. Calc. phos.*
Pain at pit of stomach, *Kali phos.*
Regurgitation, *Magnes. phos.*
Thirst, burning, *Kali sulph.*
Vomiting acid, *Nat. phos.*
" after cold water, *Calc. phos.*
" after nursing, *Silica.*
" before breakfast, *Ferr. phos.*
" bile, *Nat. sulph.*
" blood, *Ferr. phos.*
" coffee-grounds *Nat.mur.*
" infantile, *Calc. phos.*
" mucus, *Nat. mur.*
Waterbrash, *Nat. phos.*, *Kali phos.*

Abdomen and Stool.

Abdomen feels cold, *Kali sulph.*
" sunken, *Calc. phos.*
" swollen, *Kali phos.*
" tender, *Kali mur.*
" tympanitic, *Kali sulph.*

Anus, abscesses around, *Calc. sulph.*
" eruption around, *Nat. mur.*
" fissures, *Silica.*
" fistula, *Calc. phos.*
" prolapse, *Calc. sulph., Kali phos.*
" warts, *Nat. sulph.*
Burning pain, *Nat. mur.*
Colic, *Magnes. phos.*
" infantile, *Calc. phos.*
" lead, *Nat. sulph.*
Congestion of liver, *Nat. sulph.*
Constipation, alternating with diarrhea, *Nat. mur.*
" habitual, *Kali sulph.*
" in aged, *Calc. phos.*
" infantile, *Magnes. phos.*
" with furred tongue, *Kali mur.*
Cramps, *Magnes. phos.*
Diarrhea, from fatty food, *Kali mur.*
" bilious, *Nat. sulph.*
" foul, putrid, *Kali phos.*
" from chill, *Ferr. phos.*
" from fright, *Kali phos.*
" from fruit, *Calc. phos.*
" green, *Nat. phos.*
" involuntary, *Nat. mur.*
" in wet weather, *Nat. sulph.*
" painless, *Kali phos.*
" slimy, *Kali sulph.*
" undigested, *Ferr. phos.*
" watery, *Nat. mur., Magnes. phos.*
" white stools, *Nat. phos.*
" yellow stools, *Kali sulph.*
Dysentery, *Ferr. phos., Kali mur.*
Gallstones, *Calc. phos.*
" colic, *Magnes. phos.*
Hemorrhoids, *Ferr. phos., Calc. fluor.*
Itching of anus, *Nat. phos.*
Jaundice, *Kali mur., Nat. sulph.*
Liver, congested, *Nat. sulph.*
" painful, *Calc. sulph.*
Liver, soreness, *Nat. sulph.*
" torpid, *Kali mur*
Marasmus, *Calc. phos.*
Rectum, prolapse of, *Calc. sulph., Kali phos.*
" stitches in *Nat. mur.*
Worms, *Nat. phos.*
" thread, *Ferr. phos., Nat. phos.*

Urinary Symptoms.

Bladder, catarrh of, *Kali mur., Nat. mur.*
Bleeding from urethra, *Kali phos.*
Bright's disease, *Calc. phos., Kali phos.*
Burning after urinating, *Nat. mur.*
Burning during urinating, *Nat. sulph.*
Diabetes, *Nat. phos., Ferr. phos.*
Gravel, *Calc. phos., Nat. sulph.*
Incontinence, *Calc. phos.*
" while coughing, *Nat. mur.*
Increased urine, *Calc. phos.*
Kidneys, inflamed, *Kali mur.*

Retention of urine, *Magnes. phos.*
Stone in bladder, *Calc. phos.*
Suppression, *Ferr. phos.*
Urine, brick-dust sediment, *Nat. sulph.*
" copious, *Calc. phos.*
" dark color, *Kali mur., Nat. sulph.*
" gravel, *Calc. phos., Silica.*
" mucus, *Silica.*
" pungent, *Calc. fluor.*
" sand, *Nat. sulph.*
" with bile, *Nat. sulph.*
" yellow, *Kali phos.*
Wetting the bed, *Ferr. phos., Calc. phos.*

Female Symptoms.

Backache with menses, *Calc. phos.*
Bearing-down pains, *Ferr. phos., Calc. fluor.*
Burning in uterus. *Nat. mur.*
Displacements, *Calc. fluor.*
Dragging sensation *Calc. fluor.*
Dysmenorrhea, *Magnes. phos.*
" as a preventive, *Calc. phos.*
" membranous, *Magnes. phos.*
Hysterical symptoms, *Kali phos.*
Icy coldness, at menses, *Silica.*
Itching, external. *Nat. mur.*
Leucorrhea, acid, *Nat. phos.*
" acrid, *Silica.*
" creamy, *Nat. phos.*
" greenish, *Kali sulph.*
Leucorrhea, irritating, *Nat. mur.*
" itching, *Silica.*
" milky, *Kali mur.*
" mucous, *Calc. phos.*
Leucorrea, profus *Silica.*
" slimy, *Kail Sulph.*
" smarting, *Nat. Mur.*
" thick, *Kali mur.*
" watery, *Nat. mur.*
" yellow, *Kali Sulph.*
Menses, acrid, *Nat. phos.*
" black, *Kali mur.*
" bright red, *Ferr. phos.*
" clotted, *Kali mur.*
" copious, *Nat. mur.*
" corrosive, *Nat. sulph.*
" delayed, *Nat. mur.*
" every three weeks, *Ferr. phos.*
" every two weeks, *Calc. phos.*
" excessive, *Kali mur., Calc. phos.*
" frequent, *Kali mur.*
" irregular, *Kali phos.*
" long-lasting. *Calc. sulph.*
" pale, *Nat. phos.*
" premature, *Kali phos.*
" profuse, *Nat. sulph., Ferr. phos.*
" scanty, *Kali phos. Nat. mur.*
" stringy, *Magnes. phos.*
" strong odor, *Kali phos.*
" suppressed, *Calc. phos. Nat. mur.*
" with coldness, *Silica.*
" with constipation, *Nat. sulph.*
" with excitement, *Nat. phos.*

Menses with headache, *Kali sulph.*
" with melancholy, *Nat. mur.*
" with morning diarrhea, *Nat. sulph.*
" with nose bleed, *Nat. sulph.*
" with pain, *Magnes, phos.*
" with rheumatic pains, *Calc. phos.*
" with sadness, *Nat. mur.*
" with twitchings, *Calc. sulph.*
" weakness, *Calc. sulph.*
After-pains, *Kali phos., Mag. phos.*
Burning in breasts, *Calc. phos.*
Enlarged breasts, *Calc. phos.*
Knots in breasts, *Calc. fluor.*
Morning sickness, *Ferr. phos,*
Nipple crack, *Silica.*
Ovarian neuralgia, *Kali phos., Magnes. phos.*
Prolapse, *Calc. fluor.*
Sensitive parts, *Silica.*
Sterility, *Silica, Nat. phos.*
Ucerations, *Kalli mur, Silica,*
Uterine displacements, *Nat. phos*

Respiratory Organs.

Asthma *Kali sulph. Nat. sulph.*
Breathing oppressed, *Ferr. phos.*
Bronchitis, *Ferr. phos., Kali mur.*
Bronchitis, chronic. *Nat. mur.*
Bronchitis, yellow expectoration, *Kali sulph.*
Burning in chest, *Ferr. phos.*
Chest, constriction, *Magnes. phos.*
" rattling of mucus, *Kali sulph.*
" soreness, *Nat. sulph., Calc. phos.*
Congestion of lungs, *Ferr. phos.*
Cough, acute *Ferr. phos.*
" barking, *Kali mur.*
" chronic, *Calc. phos., Silica.*
" convulsive, *Magnes phos.*
" croupy, *Kali mur.*
" dry, *Ferr. phos.*
" hacking, *Calc fluor.*
" hard, *Ferr. phos.*
" in the evening, *Kali sulph.*
" loose rattling, *Kali sulph.*
" loud and noisy, *Kali mur.*
" nervous, *Magnes. phos.*
" on lying down, *Mages. phos., Calc. fluor.*
" short. *Ferr. phos.*
" spasimodic, *Magnes phos.*
" suffocative, *Calc. phos.*
" tickling, *Ferr. phos.*
" whooping, *Magnes phos.*
Croup, *Ferr. phos., Calc. sulph.*
Cropy, hoarseness, *Kali sulph.*
Expectoration, clear, *Nat. mur.*
" copious, *Silica.*
" frothy, *Nat. mur.*
" greenish, *Nat. sulph.*
" loose, *Kali sulph.*
" lumpy. *Calc. fluor.*
" mucous, *Calc. phos.*
" offensive, *Silica.*
" profuse, *Kali sulph.*

Expectoration ropy, *Nat. sulph.*
" salty, *Kali phos.*
" slimy, *Kali sulph.*
" thick, *Nat. sulph., Silica.*
" watery, *Nat. mur.*
" yellowish, *Calc. fluor. Kali phos.*

Hay fever, *Kali. phos., Nat. mur.*
Heat in chest, *Ferr. phos.*
Hectic fever, *Calc. phos. Silica.*
Hoarseness, *Ferr. phos., Kali mur.*
Larynx, painful, *Ferr, phos.*
Night sweats, *Silica. Calc. phos,*
Pain in chest, *Nat. phos.*
Pleurisy,) *Ferr, phos, Kali*
) *mur, later*
Pneumonia,) *Kali sulp, Calc, sulph,*

Heart.

Aneurism, *Calc, fluor.*
Angina pectoris, *Mangnes, phos, Kali phos,*
Blood vessels enlarged, *Calc. fluor.*
Chronic heart disease, *Silica.*
Circulation sluggish, *Kali phos.*
Hypertrophy, *Nat. mur.*
Palpitation, *Ferr. phos., Magnes. phos.*
Palpitation, with sleeplessness, *Kali phos.*
Pulse felt all over, *Nat. mur.*
" full around, *Ferr. phos.*
" intermittent, *Nat. mur., Kali phos.*
" irregular, *Kali phos.*
" rapid, *Nat. mur.*

Back and Extremities.

Aching between shoulders *Kali phos.*
" of limbs, *Calc. phos.*
Ankles pain, *Silica.*
" weak, *Nat. phos.*
Arms heavy, *Silica.*
" tired, *Nat. phos.*
Back cold, *Nat. mur.*
" crick in, *Ferr. phos.*
" pain in, *Calc. fluor.*
" soreness in, *Nat. sulph.*
Backache better lying on it, *Nat. mur.*
" worse evenings, *Kali sulph.*
" worse mornings, *Calc. phos.*
Bow-legs, *Calc. phos.*
Bunions, *Kali mur.*
Burning of feet, *Calc. sulph.*
Calves, cramps, *Calc. phos., Magnes. phos.*
Chilblains, *Kali mur.*
Coccyx painful, *Silica.*
Coldness of limbs, *Calc. phos.*
Cracking of joints, *Calc. fluor.*
Crick in back, *Ferr. phos.*
" " neck, *Nat. phos.*
Edema, *Nat. mur.*
Feet tender, *Silica.*
" swollen, *Kali mur.*
Fidgety feet, *Kali phos.*
Finger joints enlarge, *Calc. fluor.*
Ganglion, *Calc. fluor.*
Glands hardened, *Calc, fluor.*
" swollen, *Kali mur.*
Goitre, *Nat. mur., Calc. fluor.*
Gout, *Ferr. phos., Nat. sulph.*
" chronic, *Nat. phos.*

Gout, rheumatic, *Calc. phos.*
Hamstrings sore, *Nat. phos.*
Hands fall asleep, *Calc. phos.*
" get stiff, *Nat. phos.*
" hot in palms, *Ferr. phos.*
" tremble, *Nat. sulph.*
Hang nails, *Nat. mur.*, *Silica.*
Hips painful, *Kali. phos.*
Housemaid's knee, *Calc. phos.*, *Silica.*
Inflamed joints, *Ferr. phos.*, *Kali mur.*
Ingrowing toe-nails, *Silica.*
Itching of limbs, *Kali phos.*
Knees painful, *Nat. phos.*
Limbs fall asleep, *Nat. mur.*
Lumbago, *Clac. fluor.*
Muscular weakness, *Kali phos.*
Nails crippled, *Silica.*
" pain at roots, *Calc. phos.*
Neck emaciated, *Nat. mur.*
" stiff, *Ferr. phos.*
Numbness, *Calc. phos.*, *Kali phos.*
Oversensitive spine, *Silica.*
Pain goes to heart, *Nat. phos.*
" in back, *Calc. phos.*, *Ferr. phos.*
" in shin bones, *Calc. phos.*
" " shoulders, *Ferr. phos.*
" through feet, *Silica.*
Paralytic lameness, *Kali phos.*
Rheumatic fever, *Ferr. phos.*, *Kali mur.*
" fever chronic, *Calc. phos.*, *Nat, phos.*
Rheumatic fever muscular, *Ferr, phos.*
Sciatica, *Magnes, phos.*, *Kali phos.*
Shifting pains, *Kali sulph.*
Shooting pains, *Kali phos.*
Slowness to walk, *Calc. phos.*
Soles burn and itch, *Calc. sulph.*
Soreness between shoulders, *Silica,*
Stumbles easily, *Kali phos,*
Tired feeling, *Calc. fluor,*
Weakness in general, *Nat, mur.*
Wrists ache, *Nat, phos.*

Nervous Symptoms,

Alcoholism, *Magnes. phos.*
Ball sensation, *Kali phos.*
Chorea. *Magnes. phos.*, *Nat. mur.*
Contortions, *Magnes. phos.*
Convulsions, *Calc. phos.*, *Magnes, phos.*
Crawling sensation *Calc phos,*
Creeping paralysis, *Kali phos.*
Debility, *Calc. phos.*
Depression, *Kali phos.*, *Nat. mur.*
Epilepsy, *Kali mur.*, *Silica.*
Exhaustion, *Kali phos.*, *Calc. phos.*
Fears, *Kali phos.*
Gait unsteady, *Nat. phos.*
Hiccough, *Magnes. phos.*
Hysteria, *Kali phos.*, *Silica.*
Infantile paralysis, *Kali phos.*
Nervousness, *Kali phos.*
Neuralgia, congestive, *Ferr. phos.*
" congestive, inercostal, *Nat. phos.*
" congestive, obstinate, *Silica,*
Night terrors, *Kali phos.*
Squinting, from worms, *Nat. phos.*

Trembling, *Nat. phos., Calc. phos,*
Twitchings, *Magnes. phos.*
Writer's cramp, *Calc. phos.*

Sleep and Dreams,

Awakes screaming, *Kali phos.*
Cry out in sleep, *Calc. phos.*
Dreams anxious, N*at. mur.*
" lascivious, *Kali phos.*
" vivid, *Kali sulph.*
Drowsiness, *Nat. sulph.*
" in old people, *Calc, phos.*
Insomnia, *Nat. mur., Kali phos.*

Febrile Symptoms.

Ague, *Nat. sulph.*
Bilious fever, *Nat phos., Nat. sulph.*
Brain fever, *Kali phos.*
Chilliness, *Silica, Calc. phos.*
Chill in morning, *Nat mur.*
Cold sweat, *Kali sulph.*
Feet cold, *Nat. phos.*
Gastric fever, *Kali sulph.*
Hay fever, *Silica.*
Hectic fever, *Calc. sulph.*
Intermittent fever, *Nat. mur.*
Night sweats, *Calc. phos. Silica.*
Perspiration about head, *Silica.*
" cold, *Kali sulph.*
" profuse, *Kali phos.*
" sour, *Nat. phos.*
Scarlet fever, *Ferr, phos.*
Typhoid fever *Kali phos.*
Yellow fever, *Nat. sulph.*

Skin

Abscess, *Silica, Calc. sulph.*
Acne, *Kali mur.*
Barber's itch, *Magnes. phos.*
Boils, *Calc. sulph.*
Bunions, *Kali mur.*
Chaps, *Calc. fluor.*
Chilblains, *Kali phos., Silica.*
Chronic skin disease, *Nat. mur.*
Coppery spots, *Silica.*
Cracks on skin, *Calc. fluor.*
" between toes, *Nat. mur.*
Dandruff, *Kali sulph.*
Eczema, *Nat. mur. Kali. sulph.*
Erysipelas, *Kali mur. Ferr. phos.*
Fissures, *Calc. fluor.*
Freckles, *Calc. phos.*
Hair falls out, *Nat. mur. Silica.*
Hives, *Nat. phos. Kali phos.*
Insect bites, *Nat. mur.*
Irritating secretions, *Kali phos.*
Itching, *Calc. phos. Kali phos.*
Ivy poison, *Kali sulph.*
Jaundiced skin, *Nat. sulph.*
Lupus, *Calc phos. Kali mur.*
Measles, *Ferr. phos., Kali mur.*
Nodes, *Silica, Calc. fluor.*
Pimples, *Kali mur., Calc. sulph.*
Shinges, *Nat. mur., Kali mur.*
Small pox, *Kali phos., Calc. sulph.*
Wrinkled skin, *Kali phos.*

Tissue.

Anemia, *Calc. phos., Nat. mur.*
Anemia of infants, *Silica.*
Atrophy, *Calc. phos.*
Boils, *Silica, Calc. sulph.*
Bone disease, *Calc. phos. Silica.*
Bruises, *Kali mur.*
Burns, *Kali. mur., Calc. sulph.*
Cancer, *Calc. phos., Kali phos.*
Carbuncles, *Silica, Calc. sulph.*
Debility, *Kali phos.*
Dropsy, *Kali. mur., Nat. sulph.*
Emaciation, *Nat. mur., Calc. phos.*
Felons *Calc. sulph.*
Glands, *Kali mur., Silica.*
Growths, *Calc. fluor.*
Hemorrhages, *Ferr. phos., Kali mur.*
Inflammations, *Ferr. phos.*
" second stage, *Kali mur.*
Injuries, *Ferr. phos.*
Marasmus, *Calc. phos.*
Offensive discharges, *Kali phos.*
Polypi, *Calc. phos., Kali sulph,*
Proud flesh. *Silica,*
Scalds, *Kali mur.*
Secretions, albuminous, *Calc. phos.*
" greenish, *Kali sulph.*
Secretions, honey-colored, *Nat. phos.*
" offensive, *Kali phos.*
" watery, *Nat. mur.*
Sprains, *Ferr. phos.*
Suppuration, *Silica, Calc. sulph.*
Vaccination, after, *Kali mur., Silica,*
Varicose veins, *Calc. fluor.*
Wasting diseases, *Kali phos.*
